MMS Health
Recovery Guidebook

Jim Humble
with Cari Lloyd

MMS Health Recovery Guidebook, Revised Edition
by Jim Humble with Cari Lloyd

Published by
James V. Humble
contact@jimhumble.is

ISBN: 978-0-9908945-4-4

First Pre-Release Edition:	Released June 2015
Second Pre-Release Edition:	Released October 2015
First Edition:	Released October 2016
Revised Edition:	Released January 2019

Contact Email: healthrecovery@jimhumble.is

Cover Design by: Rev. Paul Beaudry and Cindy Stoe

Throughout this book you will find links to external websites which we have provided as a convenience to you, the reader. Although we have made every effort to ensure these links are accurate, up to date and relevant, we cannot take responsibility for pages maintained by external providers.

Disclaimer

Preamble

This book is filled with alternative health restoration protocols that have been found to work from the experience of grassroots efforts by many people around the world. Every individual is personally responsible for his/her decision as to whether or how they use this information, or whether or not they seek officially recognized medical attention. If you wish to apply the protocols in this book, you are taking full responsibility for your actions. You accept 100% responsibility for any and all use made of any information herein.

We do not claim, nor do we believe that these protocols heal the human body. MMS1, MMS2, bentonite clay (Aztec clay), *Aloe vera*, DMSO, and all other substances, natural or otherwise, mentioned in this book do not in any way cure or heal the body. MMS1 and MMS2 are oxidizers that destroy poisons and kill pathogens by oxidation. MMS2 (hypochlorous acid [HOCl]) is the same oxidizer that the human immune system generates in order to destroy pathogens and poisons. Bentonite clay is not a healing agent but rather it absorbs poisons and pathogens and carries them out of the body. A great deal of evidence given by the FDA, EPA and various industrial corporations prove scientifically that MMS1 (chlorine dioxide) kills and or oxidizes pathogens and poisons in food, public water systems, hospitals, and even slaughter houses. It is our belief that the same thing can and does happen in the human body.

Anecdotal evidence from thousands of people around the world indicates that there is little doubt MMS1 (chlorine dioxide), and MMS2 (when dissolved in water turns to hypochlorous acid [HOCl]) have the ability to kill pathogens and/or oxidize poisons in the human body. The FDA regulations specify that chlorine dioxide (MMS1) and calcium hypochlorite (MMS2) can be used in public water systems to purify the water, and chlorine dioxide is used to preserve vegetables, meat and other items. The human body on an average is 60-75% water. It stands to reason that chlorine dioxide can also purify the water in the body just as it does in public water systems.

Once the water of the body is purified, and many of the poisons oxidized, the body can then heal the body.

We do not claim that there is *medical proof* that any of the claims herein are true. There is however, proof for those who care to check and observe. We allude to the fact that we have anecdotal evidence. Some scientifically trained people try to discount our evidence because it is *anecdotal*. When one has three or four anecdotal confirmations that may be somewhat questionable, but when the confirmations are in the thousands upon thousands, then that changes the case. Even science tells us that when there are thousands of cases of anecdotal evidence there is likely to be some correlation.

To take or not to take MMS is a personal decision. Each individual must take responsibility for their own health. Author and co-author of this book cannot take responsibility for any adverse detoxification effects or consequences resulting from the use of any suggestions or procedures described in these pages. Please read the section, "Is It Safe to Take MMS?" on page 12.

Again, none of the protocols in this book can cure an illness, or even supply nutrients for healing the human body. We do not claim these methods cure. The protocols outlined in this book will kill most disease pathogens and oxidize various poisons in the human body. Then the body is able to heal itself.

This book is dedicated to the
many suffering people
of this world.
        Jim Humble

Acknowledgments

It would take pages to adequately express my sincere gratitude to all those who have contributed in some way to this book—whether knowingly or not. I can't find the words to sufficiently express enough appreciation, but I am confident that each one will in some way at some time—receive *payback*. When you do the right thing, it always comes back to you. Nonetheless, here I want to highlight a few individuals who deserve special thanks.

Thousands upon thousands of people in need of health recovery have been the driving force for me to document this information. I want to especially thank all those who have attended seminars and who have contributed your energy and zeal, your knowledge and experience, and your inspiration. The same thanks goes to the countless people who have written in from around the world with questions, suggestions, ideas, and testimonies of what you did that worked—my deepest gratitude and appreciation goes out to all of you.

Many thanks to those who have read this book in its pre-release state and offered suggestions. And very special thanks to the main proofreaders: DD, Jan Wallace, Daniel Bender, Manuel Catedra, and Charlotte Lackney. Thank you for all the hours put in—each of you made important contributions in your own unique way.

Thank you, Archbishop Mark Grenon and sons, Bishop Jon Grenon, and Bishop Joe Grenon, for contributing the Vaccine Procedure for overcoming vaccine injuries. In addition, Mark also developed the MMS1/DMSO Patch Protocol. You will continue to be rewarded for your tremendous work in this life and the next.

Thank you, Andreas Ludwig Kalcker, for sharing with me the idea of starting out with very low dosing of MMS, which inspired me to develop the Starting Procedure—a milestone for the use of MMS.

Clara Beltrones first created what is now known as Protocol 6 and 6 to save her daughter from an appendix operation that may have taken her life. After that experience, she used Protocol 6 and 6 to help hundreds of people. Now others around the world have helped thousands using Protocol 6 and 6. Thank you, Clara, for this tremendous contribution.

A special thanks to Rev. Paul Beaudry and Cindy Stoe who created the book cover. And an extra special thanks to Cindy Stoe for laying out this book the way we wanted it. I hope that we were not too demanding on you, Cindy. Thanks for bearing with us.

Thank you, Daniel Bender and Rev. Paul Beaudry, for contributing the illustrations in this book.

It goes without saying, thanks to Matt, for all your tech support.

And finally, but certainly not least, a big "zikomo kwambiri" to Cari, my co-author, who worked what seemed like endless hours, making sure that what I wanted to say was presented in a clear and understandable way, not to mention handling all the fine-tuning and so many details! Without Cari this book would not be. I am confident, that years from now, thousands of people will have recovered their health—and it would not have happened without Cari.

Contents

Preface

Since the discovery of the Master Mineral Solution, the awareness of MMS has continued to grow throughout the world. There is a very simple reason for this: Health is a very precious asset. More and more people have discovered that MMS can be the solution to a health problem when nothing else has worked. It should therefore be no surprise that people who have had positive results with MMS share their story with their friends, family and even publically. So, the word gets around.

Unfortunately there is much misinformation floating around regarding MMS. Much of this misinformation comes from bogus media stories that intentionally attack MMS and other alternative methods.

However, some of the misinformation also comes from well-meaning people. This is due to many reasons. Some zealous folks spread the word, but have failed to keep up-to-date with new developments; therefore they are passing on outdated information. Other would-be authorities, and/or owners of websites, for any number of reasons, simply get it wrong. Whatever the case may be, there is sufficient confusion and misinformation surrounding MMS, and this has been a major factor which has compelled me to write this book.

I have written this guidebook to help you learn the fundamentals of the Master Mineral Solution (MMS) in a clear and concise manner. From my experience, I know that most people can recover from most any disease that exists. You don't need to know every little detail of how MMS works. You just need to know how to use MMS.

This book, for example, will not teach you how to make your own MMS. It is a little like electricity. One does not need to know all the science behind how electricity works in order to benefit from it. All you need to know is how to flip a switch, and voila—the light comes on. My goal is to make it as simple as possible for any newcomer to MMS to take responsibility for his/her own health recovery—to get well, and stay well.

It's very important to understand a basic principle here and that is: *simple* is not synonymous with there is no work involved. I want to be very clear, if you are seeking health recovery, it's going to take some effort on your part. It's going to require that **you** take responsibility for your own health and well-being.

Consider that if you are in poor health, it probably took you a fair bit of time, maybe years, to get there. So you can expect it to take some time, and for sure some *work,* to get back to good health. I sometimes say that MMS can be like a magic bullet, but you have to take the necessary steps to get that bullet in motion. If you so choose the road of good health, a most precious commodity, I can guarantee that I have done everything within my power to make it not void of work, but as simple as it can be. If you will follow the **Health Recovery Plan** as outlined in these pages, you can start following the directions in this book today and possibly start seeing positive results as soon as tomorrow.

In addition, I want to point out that although as the title of this book suggests, this guidebook addresses *health recovery*, per se, it is also very much about **prevention**, and consequently **longevity**. Here is some food for thought: In today's world we are bombarded with toxins on a daily basis—there is hardly any escaping it. I have discovered over the years that many people think they are doing "OK" in the health department. They have no major illness, and no particular health condition to be concerned about that they are aware of. Yet, once they include MMS into their daily routine, they often discover a whole new world of well-being! They find they begin to shed unwanted weight, and their thinking improves—brain fog, unclear thinking, and poor concentration go out the door. They have more energy, their skin becomes smoother and takes on a special *new glow*. In short, a variety of nagging little problems they learned to live with for years vanish. Although they were doing "OK" health-wise, they are now doing all the better! So you see, MMS offers much more than one might think.

If you have a serious health issue of one kind or another from which you need to recover—this book is for you. Likewise, if your health seems to be "OK" but you would like to nevertheless achieve **optimum health,** this book is also for you. Whatever category you fit in—a basic ongoing routine with MMS can help you get healthy, *keep* you healthy, and help you maintain a good quality of life into your golden years.

For those of you who already have some understanding of MMS, you may notice there are some variations of what has already been published in my other books or posted on my websites. This volume contains the latest up-to-date information, as well as quite a bit of completely new information. It includes recent improvements that myself and others have determined through on-going use of MMS around the globe. The world of MMS is vast, and we are learning new things all the time, so be sure to periodically check for updates at:

https://jimhumble.co/

If you wish to make your own MMS rather than order online, then please purchase my book *The Master Mineral Solution of the 3rd Millennium* which has detailed instructions and many other formulas. Use this book, however, for your health recovery guidelines if you so choose.

To your health,

Jim Humble

Introduction

This book is a guide for the use of one of the most amazing health-giving mineral solutions of our time, the **Master Mineral Solution**, or MMS for short. It is produced when a simple substance taken from a mineral is mixed with any one of several food grade acids. When the two are properly combined, it produces MMS1, which is highly effective in eliminating toxins and disease pathogens in the body.

In 1996, while on a gold mining expedition in South America, I discovered that MMS quickly restored health to victims of malaria. Since that time, it has proven to restore partial or full health to hundreds of thousands of people suffering from a wide range of diseases, including cancer, diabetes, hepatitis A, B, C, Lyme disease, MRSA, multiple sclerosis, Parkinson's, Alzheimer's, HIV/AIDS, malaria, autism, infections of all kinds, arthritis, acid reflux, kidney or liver disease, aches and pains, allergies, urinary tract infections, digestive problems, high blood pressure, obesity, parasites, tumors and cysts, depression, sinus problems, eye disease, ear infections, dengue fever, skin problems, dental issues, problems with prostate (high PSA), erectile dysfunction, and many others. The MMS protocols in this book have also been used to overcome addictions to alcohol and drugs, such as heroin and others, without side effects, and the list goes on. This is by far not a comprehensive list. I know it sounds too good to be true, but according to the results we have seen from around the world, I think it's safe to say when used properly, MMS has the potential to overcome most diseases known to mankind.

The health recovery procedures given in this book are the result of 22 years of teaching people how to use MMS to recover their health. Scores of people worldwide have used and applied the principles outlined in my first books, or taught in seminars. As a result, over the years I have received a great deal of feedback, much of which has contributed to this book. The successes, even in the beginning, were far beyond anything I had ever heard of. However, what we have achieved along the way has helped us arrive at something so fantastic that very few can believe it at first, but those who try it soon discover it for themselves.

The key is to **use MMS properly.** I want to point out that prior to this time, various malady lists have circulated with advice given on how to use the MMS protocols for any one of many specific illnesses. The information on these various lists is inadequate, outdated, and sometimes wrong.

Through my years of experience, I have come to the conclusion that with MMS, there is in fact, as I sometimes say, only one MMS protocol. That protocol is the **Health Recovery Plan (HRP)** as given in this book. **This is a milestone discovery and a new concept for the use of MMS.** I have come to realize that if the 50 odd protocols outlined in this book are put together correctly and used in the proper sequence, the best results will be achieved. This is not to say that one needs to use **all** of the protocols in this book. The Health Recovery Plan (see Chapter 5) explains the steps and proper sequence to follow to recover health—**and this applies to virtually all illness and disease.** MMS is not black or white. But if you will learn and apply the principles I have outlined in the HRP, I am confident that you have a good possibility to recover your health. No matter what your problem is, get going with the Health Recovery Plan. If you follow these guidelines, and pay close attention to the signals your body is giving you, health recovery is possible.

Something of significant importance in this book is the list of the Three Golden Rules of MMS (see pages 66, 83, 84, 130). These rules are absolutely essential to the Health Recovery Plan, and I might add, these same rules can be applied to any other health recovery program that one might try. **The Health Recovery Plan, along with the Three Golden Rules of MMS, are new concepts in the MMS world which everyone should pay close attention to.**

I want to clarify a very important point. Many people naturally say "MMS cures" this or that. I've made this same statement myself from time to time in certain situations, when put on the spot, or when the words were put in my mouth, or as a matter of going with the flow of terminology that others use. In our speech and in our global society, we often blur the lines with words and their meanings. But for the record, I want to clarify here, **MMS does not cure disease**. **MMS kills pathogens and destroys (oxidizes) poisons.** When pathogens and poisons in the body are reduced or eliminated, then the body can function properly, and thereby heal. I often say, "The body heals the body". MMS helps to line things up so the body can do just that.

If you decide to put into practice what this book teaches, then I expect to hear of your health recovery. I would appreciate, (and mankind would too) hearing your testimony when you have recovered. Please share your experience so others can benefit as well. Go to:

https://mmstestimonials.co/

Chapter 1

Getting Started

Welcome to the *MMS Health Recovery Guidebook*. I truly hope this book will be of help to you, whatever your health condition may be. We have spent many long hours attempting to put this information in proper order and understandable language. Before we get started, there are some terms you must know in order to understand the world of MMS. Please familiarize yourself with the definition of terms below, and refer to this list as often as needed on your journey to health recovery.

Definition of Terms

Activation: The adding of one substance to a second substance to bring about a chemical change (reaction) of some kind. When a food acid is added to sodium chlorite in order to release chlorine dioxide, it is said to be activated.

Amber Color: When citric or hydrochloric acid is added to sodium chlorite (in the percentages mentioned in this book), after 30 seconds the drops should turn amber in color. In this book when we say *amber*, we are referring to a brown color. This can be anywhere from light to dark brown, but not yellow. The *amber* color of MMS activated drops before adding water, is much like the color of a glass amber bottle (such as is used for essential oils, various medicinal potions, or for beer bottles), when held up to the light.

Chlorine Dioxide: A chemical compound (ClO_2) taken from a naturally occurring mineral. It is used in the health recovery program of this book to destroy pathogens and neutralize poisons.

DMSO (Dimethyl Sulfoxide): A natural substance derived from wood pulp. It is a solvent that dissolves many things that water cannot dissolve, including blood clots, and thus has been known to stop strokes. It is known to have many other healing qualities of its own, as well as enhancing the effectiveness of MMS, helping to carry it deeper into the tissues.

Herxheimer Reaction: Anytime large amounts of pathogens are being killed off in the body quicker than the body is able to eliminate the toxins that the dead pathogens produce, it can cause nausea, vomiting, headaches, diarrhea or other distress, such as excessive tiredness. This is called a Herxheimer reaction and is common when going through a detoxification program, such as following the protocols in this book. Please note that although the experience may not make you *feel* particularly good, experiencing a Herxheimer reaction is usually a sign that healing is taking place. This book contains guidelines on how to ease into the process of detoxification and hopefully help one minimize the effects of a Herxheimer reaction.

Master Mineral Solution (MMS): The name of a mineral/chemical solution used to help unwell people recover their health.

Mineral: The definition of the word mineral as used in this book is taken from the third definition in the Random House Dictionary and the fourth definition in the Merriam-Webster Dictionary, which are both similar. A mineral is "any substance that is neither animal nor vegetable."

MMS: Unactivated MMS, which is a 22.4% solution of sodium chlorite ($NaClO_2$) in water. (This is made from 80% sodium chlorite powder or flakes.)

MMS1: Also referred to as *activated MMS*. (Note the added "1" to MMS.) It is MMS (sodium chlorite) plus an activator (food acid). When the two are mixed together they produce MMS1 (chlorine dioxide [ClO_2]).

Note: *Although the chemical formula for **chlorine** is "Cl", the chemical formula Cl is also found in the chemical formula for **chlorine dioxide** (ClO₂), and it is also found in the chemical formula for table salt (NaCl). Chlorine dioxide is totally different from common household bleach (sodium hypochlorite, which also has Cl in its chemical formula, NaClO) which is toxic and known to be cancer causing. Chlorine dioxide (ClO₂) is not cancer causing and has an amazing ability to destroy (through oxidation) disease-causing microorganisms that may be on or in the human body, while doing no harm to the body. Because of the chemical nature of chlorine dioxide, it destroys these microorganisms in such a manner that it is also destroyed at the same time, leaving behind only a few grains of plain table salt, discharged oxygen atoms, and dead microorganisms, which the body can easily wash out of the system.*

MMS1 Dose Drops: Anytime in this book that we refer to "drops" of MMS1 (activated MMS) we only count the actual drops of MMS (sodium chlorite). Thus although we add additional activator drops to an MMS1 dose we do not count the added activator drops when referring to the drops in the dose. For example, a 3-drop dose of MMS1 will have 3 drops of MMS and 3 drops of activator acid making actually 6 drops of liquid total, but we still only say that it is a 3-drop dose.

MMS2: Calcium hypochlorite, $Ca(ClO)_2$, when mixed with water turns into a solution of hypochlorous acid, which is an oxidizing acid that the human immune system naturally produces to destroy disease germs and clean up poisons in the system.

Pathogens: Any and all microorganisms that cause disease in its host. The host may be human, animal, plant, fungus or even another microorganism.

Sodium Chlorite: Manufactured from a chemical taken from sodium chlor**ide** (NaCl, plain salt), which is a natural mineral found in large deposits throughout the world. There are many different processes for making sodium chlor**ite** ($NaClO_2$). It cannot be done in your kitchen. It must be done in a factory. When this industrial process is completed, you have sodium chlorite ($NaClO_2$), which is the raw material for making MMS. MMS is a 22.4% solution of sodium chlorite in water.

WPS: Water Purification Solution, many of these solutions are the same formula as MMS—22.4% sodium chlorite ($NaClO_2$), in purified or distilled water.

Clarification

MMS is the general acronym term used throughout the world to indicate many of the different uses of a solution of sodium chlorite in water. Sodium chlorite is a mineral/chemical, that when mixed with a food grade acid generates chlorine dioxide. Chlorine dioxide kills diseases inside and outside of the human body, and, it is chlorine dioxide which is the active ingredient used in most of our protocols.

So, the question is sometimes posed: What is MMS? Is it sodium chlorite? Or is it chlorine dioxide? The answer is:

It is both! As I said above, the term MMS is often used as a *generic* term to describe what I have called *Miracle Mineral Solution* in the past, and what I now call the *Master Mineral Solution.* In this context one might say, "Well, it's the mineral *solution*, therefore it's chlorine dioxide." Yes, but then again, a 22.4% solution of sodium chlorite is also usually sold by the name of MMS, and is called MMS in this, and other books and websites.

In our books, and as noted above in the definition list, we refer to MMS as a 22.4% solution of sodium chlorite in water, and use the acronym MMS1 to indicate that a food acid has been added to MMS which generates a chlorine dioxide solution. Technically MMS is sodium chlorite (a 22.4% solution in water), and MMS1 is MMS plus an activator, which produces chlorine dioxide. However, in every day talk both are often simply called MMS. One might say, "It's time for my MMS dose", (meaning their **activated** MMS drops in water), or "Hand me the MMS so I can mix up my dose", meaning hand me the bottle of 22.4% sodium chlorite solution which will then be mixed with food grade acid to produce chlorine dioxide. Or, taking it further, one might say, "I have to order some MMS", which is likely to mean he/she will order a bottle of sodium chlorite 22.4%, plus a bottle of food grade acid.

There are some who refer to MMS simply as "CD" for chlorine dioxide. Personally, I'm not fond of that term because it just adds more confusion to the topic. I am going into this lengthy explanation, not with the intent to confuse, but hopefully to clarify, because the term MMS has gone far and wide and is used around the world in this general way—in my opinion, there is no stopping it. I have concluded we simply have to go with the flow.

Think of it like this—I often liken MMS to the *generic* term for coffee. One might say they like to drink coffee. But the question is raised: What type of coffee? After all, there are many types and variations of coffee and ways to make it. There is drip/filter coffee, coffee made from a French press, or a percolator or in an espresso machine, or the quick and easy instant coffee. There are a variety of coffee beans and even more varieties of coffee blends. There are all types of ways to prepare and drink coffee. One might like a Cappuccino, another a Mocha Late, another a simple Espresso, an Americano, Turkish Coffee, Irish Coffee, Vienna Coffee, Café Cubano, Caffe Latte, or a good ol' cup of Juan Valdez. The point is, often when referring to all these and many more variations of coffee, if you were going out with friends, you would be likely to say, "Let's go for coffee", but when you get to the coffee shop a variety of coffee would be ordered. In this sense, coffee is a *broad* term and the same can be said for the term, MMS.

So, when it comes to mixing up doses of MMS and using it for restoring one's health according to this book, please **diligently follow the terms for MMS as listed in the definitions above,** and know that when speaking in general terms, the acronym MMS is used in a variety of ways.

Measurements Used in This Book

The primary measurements used in this book are drops, fluid ounces, milliliters, and cups. These measurements vary slightly from country to country. For example a UK fluid ounce=28.41 milliliters, an American fluid ounce=29.57 milliliters.

Many cooking operations and even laboratories round off the above figures, and I do the same. For the sake of simplicity and because this book is written to a global audience, we have rounded off the following: 1 fluid ounce to 30 milliliters; 1/2 cup to 4 fluid ounces or 120 milliliters. (Wherever one finds ounce or ounces written in this book, we are referring to a fluid ounce or fluid ounces.)

In addition, the same is true for measuring drops. There are varying factors that weigh in to measuring a drop. In this book I have chosen to follow a general rule of thumb (based on the metric system) of 20 drops equals 1 milliliter. It is important to note that drop size may differ among different droppers, bottles with dropper caps, etc. Overall, if you are using good bottles that the drops fall easy from, one drop at a time, and the bottles do not leak, or tend to give you runaway drops—everything should be fine. If your dropper bottles do not work well, consider finding another supplier for your MMS and activator.

MMS Health Recovery Guide Legend	
MMS	unactivated MMS
MMS1	activated MMS
MMS2	calcium hypochlorite
HCl	hydrochloric acid
ml	milliliter
1 ml	20 drops
1 ounce	30 ml
1 Tablespoon	15 ml
1 teaspoon	5 ml
1/2 cup	4 ounces/120 ml
cc	cubic centimeter
1 ml	1 cc
mg	milligram

CDS and CDH

Other than MMS1, there are two other forms of MMS—CDS (Chlorine Dioxide Solution) and CDH (Chlorine Dioxide Holding). Although all three forms work in slightly different ways, all three have been successful in helping people restore their health. However, in this Guidebook we will only be referring to the original MMS—that is the formula that to date has been the most tried and proven over a longer period of time. One purpose of this book is to give you, the reader, a good foundation in the use of the Master Mineral Solution. **This basic understanding is needed in order to use all the forms of MMS.** If you get these basics down you'll be well on your way to better health. The same principles in this book can be applied to the other forms of MMS. (See Appendix A.)

Is it Safe to Take MMS?

In 22 years, since the discovery of MMS, we are not aware of anyone dying or anyone suffering permanent injuries as a result of using MMS (chlorine dioxide in a solution, which is the way it is used 99% of the time throughout the world). We only know of one recorded death (an industrial accident) caused by chlorine dioxide gas many years before MMS was discovered. This is in spite of the fact that chlorine dioxide has been used extensively to purify water, to sanitize hospital floors, to disinfect slaughter houses, and to purify vegetables, along with hundreds of other uses. More than any other single mineral/chemical, chlorine dioxide through these and other means has improved the health and lives of hundreds of millions of people worldwide and still no deaths or permanent injuries have been recorded caused by the use of chlorine dioxide in 100 years. This also includes the many millions of people who have taken MMS orally for the purpose of health restoration. Compare no deaths, except a single industrial accident not related to MMS, to the approximately 950,000 deaths caused by pharmaceutical drugs yearly, or the 15,000 deaths caused by Ibuprofen and Aspirin, in the US alone. All things considered, chlorine dioxide is one of the safest, if not the safest chemical known. For more details see:

http://www.webdc.com/pdfs/deathbymedicine.pdf

DMSO (dimethyl sulfoxide) is also used in some of our protocols. In the 60 years since DMSO was introduced in the USA there has never been a report of permanent damage or a death caused by DMSO. DMSO has been scientifically proven to have healing qualities of its own as well as enhancing the effectiveness of MMS.

What MMS is Not

There have been critics who have tried to discredit MMS by saying that it is "bleach" or it is derived from bleach, therefore I would like to explain some basics here. To *thoroughly* cover this subject, it is necessary to delve quite deeply into chemistry. However, the basics are quite simple and that is what I will touch on here. Although chlorine dioxide (ClO_2) and table salt (NaCl) both have the chlorine element in its composition (again, note the "Cl" in both formulas stands for chlorine), in this case the chlorine is in a form that is *not* dangerous and is in fact helpful. On the other hand, household bleach which is sodium **hypo**chlorite (NaClO), also has Cl in the formula, but in this case the chlorine (Cl) is in a different form and can be, in some cases, very dangerous. **(Please note that these three substances, although they all have "Cl" in some form in the formula, are all completely different.)**

You can look on the internet for the MSDS (Material Safety Data Sheet) for this information. This safety data sheet shows under "Stability Data" that sodium hypochlorite (NaClO), which again, is household bleach, can react with toilet bowl cleaners, rust removers, vinegar, acids, and ammonia products to produce hazardous gases that have caused hospitalization and even death. As many as 2,200 hospitalization incidents occur each year with British subjects. When mixed with various tap waters and brought in contact with the human body it can produce chemicals that are cancer causing, which chlorine dioxide and table salt cannot do.

Chlorine dioxide is manufactured in one of several different processes from minerals and chemicals taken from the naturally occurring mineral, sodium chloride (NaCl), which is actually table salt. So, common table salt, sodium chloride (NaCl) through various manufacturing processes becomes sodium chlorite ($NaClO_2$). Chemically this is done by adding two atoms of oxygen (O_2) to each molecule of salt (NaCl) to produce ($NaClO_2$) which is sodium chlorite. Then when this sodium chlorite is mixed with a weak food acid it becomes chlorine dioxide (ClO_2) which is the main active ingredient in the protocols discussed in this book.

Chlorine dioxide has hundreds of uses in industry and is used at more than 1,000 times stronger than the MMS Health Recovery solution in this book. Our standard dose of 3 drops of sodium chlorite solution (22.4% sodium chlorite in water) in 4 ounces/120 ml (1/2 cup) of water does not make any kind of a solution that can be called "bleach" referring to something strong enough to clean a toilet, etc. Critics that talk about MMS being bleach only succeed in unnecessarily scaring people and causing those they scare to continue suffering or even die. Just look at the formula—$NaClO_2$ (sodium chlorite/MMS) is different than NaClO (sodium hypochlorite)—different formula, different substances. So be smart, don't let others fool you!

Understanding Oxidation

Oxidation

The tiny particles of the universe are held together by the electrons that surround them. Any action that results in the change of the electrons that hold matter together is considered oxidation. You may have thought that oxidation is somehow adding oxygen to what is being oxidized, but not so. Basically, oxidation either removes or changes the position of electrons that hold things together. This either completely destroys the substances or changes them into something else.

MMS and Oxidation

MMS1 (chlorine dioxide) destroys pathogens (disease-causing microorganisms) not by using oxygen, but by oxidizing them. MMS1 draws away some of the electrons that hold the pathogens together, thus resulting in their destruction. MMS1 is also completely destroyed in the destructive process, leaving behind only a very minute amount of table salt (sodium chloride [NaCl]) and neutralized oxygen that simply washes out of the body. Various poisons created by the pathogens are also destroyed by the oxidation process. The fact is that MMS1 does not heal the body from sickness. As the oxidation process of killing the pathogen takes place, it is the body, freed from toxins, that heals the body. Beneficial bacteria are highly resistant to oxidation and thus are not harmed by chlorine dioxide.

Other Oxidizing Processes

Oxygen is the oxidizer that nature has designated for use in the human body because of its many important characteristics. Current oxygen therapies involve more than just breathing. In one type of oxygen therapy, the subject enters a pressurized hyperbaric chamber filled with pure oxygen. Pure oxygen under pressure is many times more effective than non-pressurized oxygen. This has many benefits and in some cases has worked miracles. Unfortunately, the increased pressure also multiplies the negative characteristics of oxygen, namely increasing the oxygen's ability to oxidize (destroy) good cells as well as bad ones. This treatment is also very expensive, and multiple treatments are usually required; therefore, the majority of mankind simply cannot afford the cost.

Two other very powerful oxidizers that are sometimes used in the body are hydrogen peroxide and ozone. While both of these have been and are used to help eradicate disease, at the same time, they can damage the body when used improperly. Both are more powerful than oxygen or MMS1 (chlorine dioxide). Hydrogen peroxide and ozone can and do destroy many things including human body tissues.

Pathogens hide deep in body tissues. Because hydrogen peroxide and ozone, just like chlorine dioxide, are destroyed when they oxidize something, they are usually destroyed by oxidizing body tissues before they reach the pathogens hiding in the tissues. They can also be destroyed by poisons and impurities in the blood and tissues. Ozone and hydrogen peroxide may be useful sometimes but they should never be used by someone who is not highly trained in their use.

The oxidation potentials of these four oxidizers are given below. The strength of any particular oxidizer is measured in volts and as you can see, chlorine dioxide (MMS1) is the least strong of the four oxidizers. Because MMS1 is *selective* (oxidizing pathogens and not body tissues), it can be both more effective in oxidizing pathogens, as well as being safer than these other oxidizers.

Chlorine Dioxide	0.95 volts
Oxygen	1.30 volts
Hydrogen Peroxide	1.80 volts
Ozone	2.07 volts

Note: *For a more detailed explanation of understanding MMS and the oxidation process, read the book **The Master Mineral Solution of the 3rd Millennium** Chapter 21, Oxidizers and Oxidation, and the Appendix, Understanding MMS. Read the entire book for a detailed understanding of all aspects of MMS and its function.*

A Word to the Wise

It has been my experience that some people occasionally come up with reasons to alter the techniques and protocols as explained in this book. This often hinders the protocols from working or from working as good as they can. The information in this book is the result of millions of people taking MMS over a period of 22 years. Many around the world have learned through experience that these protocols work best when followed as they are given here. So please, go by the book, follow the instructions carefully, and for optimum results, please, do not alter the procedures.

This book is chock full of essential details that are important to know in order to recover health. If you are not aware of some of these vital details it can prevent your recovery, likewise, other important points can help insure your recovery. I strongly encourage you to **read this book in its entirety**—from front to back! You do not want to cut corners when learning about MMS.

It is important to know that although I encourage you to read the complete book, **you do not have to finish the book before you get started** on the Health Recovery Plan (Chapter 5). Once you have read and understand Chapter 1 through Chapter 6, you can start on your path to health recovery, beginning with the Starting Procedure (see page 79). You don't need to know the whole book inside out to get started, but do keep reading and educate yourself on the MMS Health Recovery Plan. By reading through all of it, you will have an understanding of the various ways that MMS can be used—and you will learn some very important do's and don'ts essential to health recovery.

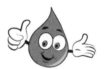

Memory Restored: An elderly guy (in his 80-90's), who claimed he was the last survivor of the chemical company (since closed), that used to operate in New Plymouth, and made Agent Orange, and many other toxic sprays. After 50 odd years working there, he said that he was so full of toxins that he couldn't remember things that he had done the day before, along with other health effects relating to a build-up of toxins in the body. Someone told him about MMS, which he tried. He phoned me on the second day all excited, saying that he remembered all he had done the day before. He claimed to be 100% better within about a week on MMS. He is now an advocate for MMS, telling everyone who is willing to listen. —P

Chapter 2

Safety Precautions

Chlorine dioxide has been used safely for a hundred years in hospitals, food preparation, water purification and for many other things. It has been used in recent times very safely by millions of people to improve their health with great results. There are, however, a few instances where caution needs to be applied. We want you to have the most pleasant experience possible while regaining your health. Do not be put off by these precautions, but be aware of them before you begin your journey to optimum health.

Some of the safety precautions listed below appear in other sections of this book under the various subjects that they pertain to. We are repeating them here, in order to give you this compiled list for your easy reference. Please note that some of the important safety measures listed below only appear on this list.

MMS/MMS1

➤ Keep MMS out of reach of children and pets. There have been no fatalities to date, however, a few children have been very sick after accidentally drinking a very large dose (not designated for a child) of MMS.

➤ Never allow MMS (sodium chlorite solution) to sit in an unmarked bottle or glass. It has no smell and it is often difficult or impossible to tell the difference between MMS and water. Some people have drunk as much as 1/2 of a glass before realizing that they were not drinking water. This is a huge overdose of undiluted, concentrated MMS, and they were in the hospital for a couple of weeks! In the case of an overdose, should a person drink too much MMS either by mistake or on purpose, they should immediately drink as much water with salt as possible to induce vomiting (use 1 tablespoon of salt per 1 liter/quart of water); then drink more salt water and try to vomit again, and do this several times. If they still feel bad after this process they should go to a hospital.

➤ Make sure all bottles of MMS, acid, etc. are clearly labeled so you can easily know what is in them. Ideally, the labels should be in different colors to make it easy to differentiate them. If using paper labels, it helps to cover them with Scotch tape, to avoid them disintegrating and falling apart, if leakage gets on them over time.

➤ I have suggested the use of a spray bottle for the eyes as well as for topical use for other body parts. However, the formula for use in the eyes is significantly different than the formula for topical skin use. Be especially careful to keep these two different spray solutions very well marked. Never use the spray bottle intended for the skin in the eyes.

➤ If you take too much MMS1 and have a serious Herxheimer reaction, (nausea, vomiting, excessive diarrhea) take Vitamin C as an antidote. Take 2 grams (2,000 mg) of Vitamin C at once. If the symptoms persist, you can then take another 1 gram of Vitamin C the following hour, and another 1 gram the third hour. Do not go over this amount of Vitamin C. Two other options to use as an antidote would be: Eat a fresh apple. Do not bite and swallow, this must be chewed very well. Or take 1 level teaspoon of bicarbonate of soda in 1/4 of a cup (2 ounces/60 ml) of water. Drink a few more sips of plain water after this if desired.

➤ If your home has a septic tank do not dump MMS waste down the drain as it can kill the bacteria in your tank. This makes a mess and is expensive to repair.

➤ MMS liquid full strength out of the bottle (22.4% sodium chlorite solution) can irritate the skin. If it comes into direct contact with the skin, rinse it off with clean water. Try to avoid getting it on clothes as the concentrated solution can discolor them. A dilute solution may also discolor some fabrics, depending on the concentration and the fabric. (There are two exceptions to this rule of putting full strength MMS on the skin, you can do so for short periods of time to help burns and mosquito bites, see pages 245 and 196 for proper instructions.)

➤ Avoid breathing in high concentrations of chlorine dioxide gas produced from the mixing of sodium chlorite and an acid activator. Chlorine dioxide gas easily escapes when MMS and activator are mixed and are not in a sealed container. It is best to avoid getting a direct whiff of it as it could cause coughing. Do not mix your dose directly under your nose or mouth. If doing the Bag Protocol, (see page 156) be especially careful not to directly breathe in the fumes. There are times when breathing in the gas in small controlled amounts (see page 159) are called for and it can be very healing to the lungs and sinuses, but do avoid this unless you are under a specific protocol requiring it and know what you are doing, as it is easy to inhale too much.

➤ MMS protocols have been known to cancel out the effect of birth control pills.

➤ When traveling with, or transporting MMS, activator acid, and other supplies necessary to do the protocols in this book, be sure to separate all the different types of liquids and powders. MMS (sodium chlorite) and the acid activator should be packed separately, never in the same bag, so as to avoid spills and possible premature activation. **DMSO should never, ever be packed in the same container or suitcase as MMS2** (see important warning on page 26). Be sure that all these are properly packaged so they cannot possibly spill. (Suggestion: Put in plastic bags, tape, and then put in double Ziploc bags.) If traveling by air, be sure to know the airline regulations for transporting various types of liquids and supplies (and in what quantities) on the carrier that you are using. Be responsible and diligent to carefully pack to avoid any problems for yourself or others, or reflect negatively on MMS in general.

CALCIUM HYPOCHLORITE (MMS2)

➤ Calcium hypochlorite can ignite with even a very small spark when it comes in contact with organic materials. For example: if someone stuffed a rag (any type of cloth) down into the calcium hypochlorite jar and for any reason a spark from a candle, cigarette, or any other kind of spark hit it, it would cause an instant and extremely hot fire.

➤ In case of a spill of calcium hypochlorite powder, clean it up with two dustpans, or one dustpan and a wet rag, but do not use a broom, because a spark could easily ignite the broom when in contact with the calcium hypochlorite powder.

➤ Calcium hypochlorite is hygroscopic and will draw moisture from the air. If your supply becomes moist, discard it, but not down the drain if you have a septic tank. If you have a city sewer a small amount, about a liter, will not hurt it. You can discard it in a city dump, or with a city trash collector, after adding a small amount of water to it to insure that it cannot ignite.

➤ Avoid contact with skin and eyes when in the powder form.

➤ Do not directly breathe the fumes from calcium hypochlorite.

➤ Do not make more MMS2 capsules than you need for a month, as the capsules will become brittle and can easily break open.

➤ If you use a capsule machine to make up your MMS2 capsules (see pages 93-94, 274-278), use one that is made from plastic, as the calcium hypochlorite powder should not come into contact with metal.

WARNING

- Do not allow calcium hypochlorite (MMS2) to come into contact with DMSO. This will cause immediate combustion with extreme heat and fire. In this case, it does not need a spark to start the fire instantly. Use water to put out such a fire but stand back as the water will spatter.

- Calcium hypochlorite (MMS2) should never, ever be packed in the same container, box, or suitcase as DMSO. When transporting these items **always pack them separately.**

INGESTION WARNING

- Never use DMSO in a drink while at the same time taking calcium hypochlorite (MMS2) capsules. The DMSO can cause the MMS2 to heat and it could become very uncomfortable in your stomach. (If this should happen by accident, drink plenty of cold water to alleviate any discomfort.)

- If adding DMSO to an MMS1 dose, as per Protocol 1000 Plus for example, you must calculate no more than 3 drops of DMSO per each drop of MMS1, and it must be mixed in at least 1/2 cup (4 ounces/120 ml) of water.

- If on a protocol that calls for taking MMS2 in the same day as MMS1/DMSO doses, you can do this, but the MMS2 capsule must be separated out by one-half hour from the MMS1/DMSO doses. **Never take a dose of anything containing DMSO and an MMS2 capsule at the same time!**

CITRIC ACID/HYDROCHLORIC ACID (HCl)

➤ Citric acid and hydrochloric acid (HCl) on their own, should not come into contact with the skin. The acid can be washed off the skin with clean water. If the acid gets into the eyes, wash the eye with clean water until the stinging feeling is gone. If you wash the eye immediately, there should be no problem, but if you take as long as 30 seconds before getting clean water into your eye, there may be a problem and you should go to an emergency clinic right away, but not before rinsing the eye thoroughly with water. Some suggested precautions to avoid splashes in the eyes to begin with would be—wear glasses when pouring acids, take care to keep the bottle at a distance and height so as to avoid a splash in the eye, use a deep enough glass.

➤ For some (not all) people, citric acid has been known to cause significant stomach upset. Should this be the case, use 4% HCl as an activator for MMS instead of citric acid.

➤ Our protocols call for 4% HCl. In this concentration it should not do serious damage if accidentally spilled on the skin, but it should, nevertheless, be rinsed off immediately.

However, higher strength HCl and other high strength acids can be harmful if not handled properly. Keep in mind that anytime you transport or carry strong acids any distance further than within the same room, you should also carry water with you. This will enable you to immediately rinse any spilled acid off of your skin or out of the eyes. Large spills can cause severe damage and even death if not rinsed off the skin or out of the eyes immediately. In the event you need to handle HCl in a high concentration, do so in a very well ventilated area, use a proper mask, wear gloves and be very careful to not breathe in the fumes, as it can cause damage.

DMSO

➤ DMSO is a solvent, and easily passes through the skin and into the tissues. It will also carry other substances along with it, so be careful what you have on the skin before handling DMSO.

➤ If applying DMSO topically, be sure your hands and nails are clean and free from contaminants (including soap residue) when handling DMSO. You want to also be sure the area to which you *apply* DMSO is clean.

➤ When washing an area of the skin *before* applying DMSO, it is best, if possible, to use natural, chemical-free soap to wash application areas and hands. Whether this is available or not, be sure any soap is *completely* rinsed off—or use no soap at all. Simply wash well (rubbing the skin) with clean water.

➤ The best method to apply DMSO to the skin is simply to use clean dry bare hands when rubbing the DMSO into your body or on someone else.

➤ If using bare hands to apply DMSO, do not wear finger nail polish. DMSO is a solvent that will not only dissolve the polish, but will also carry its toxic ingredients through the skin and into the body. You can cover your hand in a plastic sandwich bag (this type of plastic in general, is OK for use with DMSO) to apply the DMSO.

➤ After handling DMSO, *never wash it off* with soap as it can carry the soap into the skin/tissues. Simply rinse the hands well with clean water.

➤ Keep full strength DMSO out of your eyes.

➤ Do not use most common gloves (rubber, latex, etc.) with DMSO. It can dissolve the gloves. Even dissolving a tiny bit of the gloves can then transfer the rubber or latex into your body. Gloves made of non-stretchable plastic are OK to use with DMSO. Normally DMSO will not hurt one's hands, and gloves are not needed. (If applying frequently or in large amounts for some skin types it may cause the skin to become wrinkly, but this soon passes.)

➤ **Never add DMSO to an enema solution**. The colon contains many toxins the body is flushing out. If you put DMSO in the colon, you can return some of those toxins back into the blood stream.

WARNING

- Do not allow DMSO to come into contact with calcium hypochlorite (MMS2). This will cause immediate combustion with extreme heat and fire. In this case, it does not need a spark to start the fire instantly. Use water to put out such a fire but stand back as the water will spatter.

- DMSO should never, ever be packed in the same container, box, or suitcase as calcium hypochlorite (MMS2). When transporting these items **always pack them separately.**

INGESTION WARNING

- Never use DMSO in a drink while at the same time taking calcium hypochlorite (MMS2) capsules. The DMSO can cause the MMS2 to heat and it could become very uncomfortable in your stomach. (If this should happen by accident, drink plenty of cold water to alleviate any discomfort.)

- If adding DMSO to an MMS1 dose, as per Protocol 1000 Plus for example, you must calculate no more than 3 drops of DMSO to each drop of MMS1, and it must be mixed with at least 1/2 cup (4 ounces/120 ml) of water.

- If on a protocol that calls for taking MMS2 in the same day as MMS1/DMSO doses, you can do this, but the MMS2 capsule must be separated out by one-half hour from the MMS1/DMSO doses. **Never take a dose containing DMSO and an MMS2 capsule at the same time!**

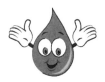

Heroine Free: Thank you for giving our world MMS. I have personally helped quite a few people to get off a full blown heroin addiction in three to four days only with 3/4 drop of MMS1 an hour. This is every hour when they are awake. I have also included MMS1 baths, using 25 drops of MMS1 per bath. I have personally assisted a hand full of people with 100% unbelievable results. —Ravi, England

Candida Gone: I had Candida so badly that not only was I exhausted for years on end, but the fungus had migrated to my eyes and ears. It was like looking out through sheets of waxed paper. My ears buzzed and rang non-stop. I itched all over, especially at night when it was so bad it would wake me from a deep sleep. I had many other symptoms and tried many cures, none of which worked until I tried MMS. I had to change my diet to a very low carb diet because sugar feeds yeast. I don't think you can get better if you continue eating the standard American diet, so I modified my diet to include almost no grains, no sugars of any kind, and very limited fruit. You must do this in order to recover. I had found a product called Syclovir that did a great job at holding the symptoms at bay, but there was no cure even after a year on the product. Then I read that MMS could help kill Candida so I took 7 drops 4 times per day and began to see improvement. I think it's been about 2 months of this approach and my energy is sky high. I can tolerate more carbs now with no symptoms. I feel great and I know it's because of the MMS. In addition, MMS has reversed the arthritis I had in my toes and it must have cleaned out my veins because I can now exert myself and not become out of breath. What a miracle MMS has proved to be in my life! —Kathryn

Multiple Recoveries: MMS1 and 2 has cured me of prostate enlargement/pain...gum/tooth infection and candida. Amazing! I use MMS to bathe in...great for the skin and tired muscles. —James A., New Zealand

Chapter 3

MMS Basic Essentials

There is some fundamental information which you must know before attempting to use MMS. Like many things, MMS is easy to use once you are familiar with it. But, the last thing you should do is try to use it without knowing what you are doing. If you choose to take responsibility for your own health, please do your homework before attempting to carry out any of the protocols in this book.

Here are two key factors that could make a world of difference to your health recovery:

1. Every time you start a protocol, even though you may have read the book initially or some months back, be sure to thoroughly review the information in the particular protocol you are about to begin. It is important to **have a clear understanding of everything that must be done *before* starting.** This will help you gather all the materials needed for the protocol, and help you avoid getting to a certain step in the protocol and being caught short, or realizing you did something wrong in the beginning. Some protocols are more detailed than others and some contain important cautions and/or details that are essential to success. So refresh your memory and have a clear understanding of every detail before you begin a protocol.

2. If at all possible, have a partner. MMS has many uses. You may do just fine using a protocol for a general cleanse

or to overcome a common cold. But when you are very sick, whether it be with a very bad flu or a more serious or long term illness, you may not feel up to mixing a dose, or preparing a bath or keeping track of hours and measurements. Don't try to go it alone. Find someone, a spouse, a parent, son or daughter, aunt or uncle, grandparent, a friend or a caregiver, who can help you on your journey to wellness.

Activating MMS

Citric Acid and Hydrochloric Acid (HCl)

MMS needs a food-grade acid to "activate it" and the two combined produce MMS1 (chlorine dioxide). There are several acids that can activate MMS, including the juice of a fresh lemon or lime, or vinegar. However, in this book when we refer to using an acid to activate MMS we mean using either 50% citric acid, or 4% HCl (hydrochloric acid). When using these two acids in these percentages always use 1 drop of acid to 1 drop of MMS. Both of these acids, in these percentages, are a 1-to-1 ratio with MMS. In other words, mix 1 drop of either of these acids to every 1 drop of MMS. The standard activation time for mixing these drop-for-drop doses using 50% citric acid or 4% HCl is 30 seconds. See page 32 for full instructions on how to mix a basic MMS1 dose.

We prefer HCl as the **activator of choice** because it is the same acid that is produced naturally in your stomach. Many people consider it has a better taste and is easier on the stomach.

Some Alternative Acids

Both citric and hydrochloric acid are easy to use as activators for MMS; however, depending on your location and availability, or in an emergency, other activators such as fresh lemon or lime juice, or vinegar, can be used to activate MMS but they measure differently. If using any of these acids, you will need to use 5 drops of lemon, lime or vinegar for every 1 drop of MMS, at a 1-to-5 ratio. If using these alternative acids, activation time must be three minutes, instead of 30 seconds which is the standard activation time for either 50% citric acid or 4% HCl.

Notes

➤ *When using the juice of a fresh lemon or lime it is important to not use a citrus press that in any way squeezes the peel (skin or outer surface) of the lemon or lime. The properties of the oil from the lemon/lime peel if mixed with the juice can prevent the activation of sodium chlorite and thus leave one with a dose that is useless. You can prevent this problem by squeezing the lemon/lime by hand. The various plastic and metal squeezers (especially the hand held type) put too much of the peel's oils into the juice of the lemon/lime. So squeeze the lemon/lime by hand. By this I mean cut the lemon/lime in half, take one half into your hand and gently squeeze out the number of drops you need. Simply count the drops as they fall for the amount of drops you need for your dose.*

➤ *Never use ascorbic acid, or hydrofluoric acid; because ascorbic acid will neutralize the MMS and hydrofluoric acid is extremely poisonous.*

➤ *Throughout this book we suggest using 50% citric acid as an activator. This has been used for years with success in MMS formulas. There are some however, who use 33% or 35% citric acid. Availability in different percentages varies from country to country. These percentages are also acceptable to use for mixing up a dose of MMS1. At these percentages (33% and 35% citric acid), you also use a 1-to-1 drop ratio with MMS and wait 30 seconds for activation time.*

Mixing a Basic Dose of MMS1

Various protocols are discussed in this book. These use varying numbers of drops depending on several factors. Here we will only discuss the basic concept of mixing.

Step 1

❑ Always use an empty, clean, dry, drinking glass.

❑ Tilt the glass slightly sideways and drop your drops of MMS so they go to the corner of the bottom part of the glass. Always hold the dropper bottle or pipette (eye dropper) straight up and down when dropping drops.

❑ If using a 50% solution of citric acid or 4% solution of HCl, add the same amount of activator on top of the MMS drops. (For each drop of MMS add 1 drop of acid.)

Step 2

❑ Swirl the drops a little as you count to 30 seconds; in this amount of time the mixture should turn amber in color.

Step 3

❑ Then add 1/2 cup (4 ounces/120 ml) of drinking water or juice or other liquid as per the instructions on pages 41-45.

❑ Drink your dose while fresh, in less than one minute.

Mixing a Basic Dose of MMS1

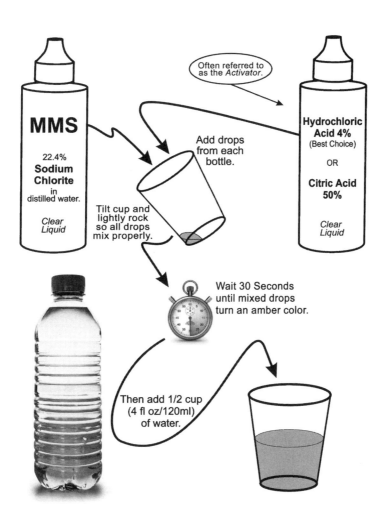

MMS
22.4%
Sodium
Chlorite
in
distilled water.

Clear
Liquid

Often referred to
as the *Activator*.

Hydrochloric
Acid 4%
(Best Choice)

OR

Citric Acid
50%

Clear
Liquid

Add drops
from each
bottle.

Tilt cup and
lightly rock
so all drops
mix properly.

Wait 30 Seconds
until mixed drops
turn an amber color.

Then add 1/2 cup
(4 fl oz/120ml)
of water.

Be careful: Some chlorine dioxide gas is likely to escape when MMS and activator are mixed and are not in a sealed container. It is best to avoid getting a direct whiff of it. Do not mix your dose directly under your nose or mouth. There are times when breathing in the gas in small amounts is called for and it can be very healing to the lungs and sinuses, but avoid this unless you are under a specific protocol requiring it and know what you are doing, (as it is easy to inhale too much).

Hourly Doses

When I wrote my first book, I instructed people to work up to 3 large doses of MMS1 each day. If you read my first book, or any one of a number of random web sites that have put up information from that book, and unfortunately have not updated it, then it is time to learn something new. In the beginning, when I suggested the larger dose, I always had people *work up* to it a little at a time. Back then the suggestion was to work up to a 15-drop dose taken 3 times a day.

The drawback of the old method was that many people were having a pretty strong Herxheimer reaction. They would feel a lot worse before they got better. With time, and with more experience under my belt, I began to realize that taking smaller doses of MMS1 more often throughout the day brought better results. Perhaps the most important reason for this is because MMS1 only lasts in your system for an hour, possibly an hour and a half at most. So keeping MMS1 running through your system on an hourly basis is imperative. This way MMS1 is hitting the pathogens continuously and does not allow pathogens time to regroup and build back up. Instead, being constantly hit without a chance to regroup, they die off. This new method works and we clearly see positive results.

In 2009, I went to Malawi, a small country in southeast Africa. While there, 800 HIV/AIDS cases came to me. These people took only 3 drops of MMS1 every hour, for eight hours a day, for three weeks. Guess what? The 3-drop doses, taken eight hours a day for 21 days, were 99% effective in eradicating HIV/AIDS. There were only five failures out of the 800 cases, and of these five, instructions were not properly followed in one way or another.

Since that time hundreds of thousands of people have taken 3–drop doses on an hourly basis and have recovered their health. This change to smaller hourly doses, as opposed to large doses less often, probably represents the biggest development from earlier instructions.

To sum it up, after years of experience, we have come to learn that most diseases (other than malaria), are substantially more responsive to **hourly doses** of MMS1, spread out over an eight to ten hour period daily. This is more effective than 1, 2, or 3 large doses per day. This is true for cancer and for most diseases. People have been using hourly protocols in recent years with amazing success. There are a few other exceptions to the hourly dose rule, other than malaria, such as Protocol 6 and 6 (see page 169), and some of the Emergency Protocols (see Chapter 12).

So, to reiterate: **Please do not follow instructions that talk about 3 large doses of 15 drops each.** (Unless it is an exception to the rule, as mentioned above.)

The Importance of Consecutive Doses

Be diligent to take your dose consecutively every hour on the hour. For example, while on an eight-hour protocol, do not break up your dosing hours such as four hours in the morning, then a three hour break, then four more hours later in the day.

> A fundamental principle of MMS is that hitting the pathogens every hour does not give pathogens time to regroup and build back up, but instead, being constantly hit without a chance to regroup, they die off.

Daily Dose Bottle

In recent years we have taught the use of a *daily dose bottle*. The main inspiration for this bottle was to help facilitate people in taking their *hourly* dose. However, we have since concluded that **maximum benefit from taking MMS1 is derived when each hourly dose is made up fresh**. This phenomenon was first noticed with thousands of autistic children who used the daily dose bottle for an ample time period. Then, when the children were switched over to doses made up individually and fresh each hour, many more improvements were reported than when their doses were mixed into one bottle for the entire day.

In my 22 years of working with MMS, and personally helping thousands of people, I have noticed overall *greater* results in health recovery when individually mixed fresh doses of MMS1 were used. In addition, our very active Health Ministers around the globe who work extensively with MMS, and with large numbers of people (by the thousands), have also reported the same results.

If for various reasons there is no other choice but to make up an all-day mixture instead of mixing each dose fresh every hour, it is certainly well worth your while, and better than taking no MMS at all. But my recommendation is, if at all possible, stick to mixing fresh hourly doses. You will have a greater chance of getting well much quicker.

Note: *A daily dose bottle entails mixing up all your MMS1 doses for the day into one bottle from which you drink a certain amount each hour. For example, if you were on Protocol 1000, it calls for taking a 3-drop dose of MMS1 (3 drops is the maximum—you start with less), every hour for eight consecutive hours. If making a daily bottle you would activate 24 drops of MMS, and add the drops to a 1 liter/quart bottle of purified water. If you drink 4 ounces out of the bottle, you would have a 3-drop dose.*

There can be any number of reasons why making up a *fresh hourly dose* of MMS1 may seem challenging and not possible. Perhaps one has a job where they drive a lot. Mixing a dose while driving is not easy, nor do I recommend it. I have found, however, through receiving substantial feedback from people around the world, that where there is a will, there is a way. Consider that your health is worth the effort to find a way to mix up your hourly doses. It can be as simple as carrying your MMS and activator acid bottles around in a Ziploc bag.

Tips

➤   When you are on the go, you might want to have small 1/2 ounce (15 ml) size bottles of MMS and acid activator to carry in your purse or pocket. (These can be refilled when needed from your larger bottles at home.)

➤   If you are on the go and find yourself in and out of the office, the car, meetings, stuck in traffic and so on, purchasing a small portable pouch or lunch bag to keep your MMS supplies on hand and ready to go along with you at all times can be of help. All you need are your bottles of MMS and acid activator, a small 4 ounce/120 ml size glass, and a bottle or two of purified water. As a rule,

I do not recommend mixing and drinking your doses in plastic cups, glass is preferred. But if you are on the go, it may be convenient to take along small disposable plastic cups, 4 ounce/120 ml size. This would not be what you use all the time, but when you are on the go it could be helpful.

➤ If and when it is still not convenient to do all of the above, and you find yourself in situations where stopping to mix your dose is not possible, an alternative to succumbing to using an *all day dose bottle* as a rule rather than the exception, would be to only pre-mix doses for the hours when there is no other choice.

For example, say you are a teacher and you have to stand in front of your class for two or three hours. You know in advance you cannot excuse yourself to go mix up a dose during that time. In this case, mix up 2 or 3 doses in a bottle beforehand. Drink your hourly dose from that bottle during the time you cannot slip away to mix up a fresh dose. In almost any situation it is acceptable to have a *water bottle* on hand. Then, when possible, go back to mixing your fresh hourly doses. This helps one be able to continue with consecutive hourly doses, without breaking the 8 or 10 hour cycle of the protocols. All MMS1 doses are usually taken in 4 ounces/120 ml of water (or other compatible liquid). Try to find 4 ounce/120 ml bottles and pre-mix the amount of doses you will need, in individual bottles. Or, if you know you need two hours worth of pre-mixed doses, an 8 ounce/240 ml bottle would do, or for three hours a 12 ounce/360 ml bottle. You may want to use an indelible marking pen to mark off your bottle in 4 ounce/120 ml sections. Find what works best for you.

This method is a combination of the pre-made dose bottle and mixing up fresh hourly doses. Remember, fresh mixed doses are best, but resort to this combination of the two—fresh doses and doses prepared ahead of time in a bottle, when there is no other choice. Keeping up with consecutive hourly doses is important.

How to Test That Your MMS is Good

When activating MMS, it is very important that the drops of MMS and activator turn amber color within the first 30 seconds. In this book when we say *amber*, we are referring to a brown color. This can be anywhere from light to dark brown, but not yellow. The *amber* color of MMS activated drops before adding water, is much like the color of a glass amber bottle (such as is used for essential oils, various medicinal potions, or for beer bottles), when held up to the light.

Mix up a 3-drop dose of MMS1 to do this test, if you use less drops it will be difficult to adequately judge the color. It is best to carry out this test in a room with good lighting. When you have mixed your drops (before adding water), hold the glass up against a white or light colored background and look through the side and bottom of the glass (where your drops are) with the glass level with your eyes; at this angle you will be looking through your drop mixture. If you look *down* into the glass, the drops will often look lighter yellow, but if you view the drops at eye level (with good lighting) you should see a darker shade—that is, amber. Although it turns dark, it must also be transparent (see-through). The drops must appear amber in color. The amber color will fade and become light yellow in about 15 minutes. Do not let the solution sit for more than a minute before consuming it, as it will lose potency.

The amber color is an important indicator that the drop mixture is correct. You are mixing two clear liquids, MMS and an activator. If the liquids are mixed according to instructions they will change color and turn to amber. This amber color indicates that you have the correct liquids and a correct mixture. Very few two clear liquids can produce this same color.

If your drops do not turn amber within the first 30 seconds of mixing, something is wrong with your MMS and/or with your acid, and this mixture may not bring the desired results. You might try mixing up a dose one more time, to be sure you did it correctly, but if you still get light yellow and not amber color, you can use those drops for the time being, while you try to get some good MMS and acid activator. But I would suggest you do not use this solution (light yellow, not amber, drops) for more than a week or so. **If the solution does not at least turn yellow do not use it at all.**

Various factors can weigh in as to the color of the drops, such as the type of glass you are using, making sure the glass is completely dry to start, the number of drops you are mixing, the background color of the wall, the time of day and how much natural light is in the room and so on. If you are not getting the right color, and you are sure you have followed the directions correctly, try mixing up the drops a few times in different conditions. For example, use a different glass (some glass qualities distort) make sure the glass is clean enough—no dish soap deposits. Hold your drops up against a white wall, a white fridge, or a light background when testing the color. If in doubt of the color, mix up a 6-drop dose when testing. Test your drops under various conditions, before determining your drops are insufficient.

Note: *If you are using an alternative acid such as lemon, lime, or vinegar at a 1-to-5 drop ratio with MMS, your drops will not turn amber in color. In this case, if you want to test that the MMS is good, mix up a 3-drop dose of MMS1 (this would be 3 drops of MMS and 15 drops of lemon, lime or vinegar) and wait three minutes. Then add*

1/2 cup (4 ounces/120 ml) of water and test the ppm, which should be 25 ppm. (For testing the ppm, see page 278.)

Water—The Ideal Liquid for Mixing an MMS1 Dose

➤ The ideal is to take your MMS1 dose in water only. MMS1 doses should be taken in 1/2 cup of water (this is 4 ounces or 120 ml), or mineral water. Children usually need less than a half cup of water. When a child takes 1 drop of MMS1 or less, he should use 1/4 cup of liquid.

➤ MMS1 should be taken in drinking (purified) water— **never tap water** that has chlorine, fluoride or other toxins added, as these will cancel out the effectiveness of MMS1 and may even make you sick. Usually it is best to purchase bottled water. Keep in mind, all bottled water is not created equal. Don't automatically assume just because it's bottled, it is more safe, clean or pure than tap water. Some bottled water contains fluoride, chlorine or other harmful substances. So check out your water source. Read the labels and/or check with manufacturers to know what you are getting. Distilled water or reverse osmosis water can also be used.

Caution: Please remember that most places in the world use a toxic form of chlorine as a water purifier. Even worse than that, many places add extremely poisonous fluoride to the water because sadly, around 50 years ago doctors convinced the public that fluoride helps teeth. Fluoride is one of the most poisonous chemicals known to man. There is no evidence that it helps one's teeth and there are hundreds of thousands of teenagers who have teeth with blotches as a result. Use a good quality bottled drinking water for these protocols unless you get your water from a pure water spring or well or you have a reverse osmosis water filter. Distilled water can also be used.

Taste Factor/How to Improve the Taste of MMS1

➤ Why do MMS1 doses taste extremely bad for some people? We have noticed that some people develop extreme revulsion to taking MMS1 at one time or another while on an MMS protocol. Sometimes it gets so bad that people simply cannot take it anymore. I think there may be an explanation. Possibly the pathogens create the aversion to MMS1 as a survival mechanism for the pathogens to keep the person involved from continuing to take whatever it is that might destroy them. In any case, if this happens to you, it is well worth your while to do whatever you can to try and overcome the aversion to taking MMS1. Endeavoring to keep a positive attitude can help, then try one or some of the things mentioned below to help overcome the taste problem.

➤ Many people agree, that MMS1 doses activated with 4% HCl (hydrochloric acid) taste better than those activated with 50% citric acid. If you are using citric acid and the taste is bothersome, try switching to HCl. It is really a personal matter—see what works best for you.

➤ Though water is the ideal, if you cannot take MMS1 with water only, because the taste bothers you, some (not all) natural juices are OK to use if they do not have harmful preservatives and/or added Vitamin C or ascorbic acid, as this will cancel out the effectiveness of MMS1. Fresh juice is best. We have found apple, grape, and cranberry juice to work well with MMS1, but again, it should be natural, without preservatives and have no added Vitamin C (or ascorbic acid). Never use orange or tangerine juice in any form with MMS1. You may have these juices at least two hours before or after your MMS1 protocol for the day.

➤ Many teas are not compatible with MMS. However, there are some herbal teas that are compatible. This can vary depending on what tea you are using, i.e. the *fresh herb* or a *tea bag* that possibly is laced with a contaminant of some kind. Use the test strip method described on page 278 to be sure what is compatible.

➤ Some sodas work fine with MMS1: Coke, Pepsi, Sprite, 7-Up, and Canada Dry Ginger Ale (use only the original formulas; do not use Diet Soda or "Light" or "Zero"). We do not recommend using these drinks in the long term, or for Protocol 1000 (due to the sugar content), as you'll be drinking this 8 times a day. I would suggest fizzy mineral water as a better choice because it is sugar free. However, if taste is an issue, for someone who is seriously sick, taking an MMS1 dose in soda is better than not taking it at all. You could mix your dose in a 4 ounce/120 ml size cup and add 1 ounce of Pepsi for example, and the rest water—that may be enough soda to just cover the taste of MMS. But in many cases mineral water alone (with fizz and no sugar) helps overcome the taste.

Note: *Although I have personally tested these drinks with MMS many times, it has been brought to my attention that soda companies tend to adjust their formulas from time to time, and often differ from country to country. The safest way to know if your drink is compatible with MMS1, is to test the drink with a chlorine dioxide test strip. (See page 278 for more information on these test strips produced by the LaMotte Company, and how to use them to test compatibility with MMS1 and various liquids.) If test strips are not available and a person is on a protocol using a particular soft drink or bottled juice as a mixer, but not getting any results after five or six days, I strongly suggest switching to another liquid to drink your dose.*

➤ Smell can have a huge affect on taste. If you find you can't stomach the taste of MMS1, try changing how you drink your dose. Some people actually hold their nose while drinking their dose. A small-mouth bottle or glass, as opposed to a wide-mouth one can work wonders. Using a small-mouth bottle does not allow your nose to be inside the container that is out-gassing chlorine dioxide (ClO_2). Glasses and bottles come in all shapes and sizes. Be inventive! Be on the outlook—an empty juice bottle or jar from some other product might serve you well. Search out what works just right for you.

➤ If you would like to branch out and use various juices, or sodas other than those mentioned in this book to mix with MMS1, as a rule it is a good idea to test for compatibility with MMS. Use the test strip mentioned earlier in this section (see directions on page 278).

➤ Some people have suggested the use of stevia to improve the taste of their MMS1 drinks. We have found that the quality of stevia varies. Some is highly processed and some brands/types cancel out the effectiveness of MMS1. If you want to use stevia, we suggest you use test strips (see page 278) to confirm if the type you are using is compatible with MMS1. (A company called SweetLeaf® makes liquid stevia and their plain *non-flavored* SteviaClear® drops are compatible with MMS1. If you want to use the various flavors of SweetLeaf® stevia, again, use the test strips to be sure it's compatible with MMS1—compatibility may vary from flavor to flavor.)

➤ We personally have made up a water jug with purified water and a little honey and kept this in the fridge to mix with MMS1 drinks throughout the day. This has helped the taste to some people's liking. We do suggest however, because there are many different qualities and types of honey, (and some honey is quite adulterated) that again, the safest thing to do would be to test your drink with honey water. Use the test strip method, to be sure the type of honey you are using is compatible with MMS1.

➤ Another way to improve the taste of an MMS1 dose is to use cold water in each dose. Simply keep a bottle of purified water in the fridge for this purpose.

➤ Whatever you choose to mix with MMS1, try to drink it right away so that no more than 60 seconds passes from the time you first began mixing.

MMS1 in a Capsule (to Eliminate Taste)

Another method of taking MMS1 drops which helps elimi-nate the taste is using vegetable or gel capsules.

Step 1

❑ Have your supplies on hand. For this method you will need empty capsules and an eye dropper in addition to your drops, and a clean, dry glass for activating them. You will also need drinking water nearby to be able to take your capsule immediately after it is made. See the chart on page 46 for the proper size capsules to use for the dose you are taking.

Step 2

❑ Activate the correct amount of drops for your dose in a glass and count 30 seconds.

❑ Immediately take the eye dropper, suck up the activated drops from the glass, and carefully put them in the capsule.

❑ Push the capsule lid closed and double check it is securely in place.

Step 3

❑ Take the capsule with at least 1/2 cup (4 ounces/120 ml) of water immediately. Do not wait after filling the capsule, as the drops will begin to melt it.

Notes

➤ ***Do not activate the MMS in the capsule itself.*** *Pressure generated inside the small space of the capsule during the activation process could cause the capsule to come apart as you swallow it. So be sure to always activate the drops in a clean glass and count 30 seconds before putting the activated drops into the capsule.*

➤ *The size capsule you will need depends on the size dose you want to take. (See chart below.) Keep in mind that if you are preparing a 3-drop dose to put in a capsule, it will actually be twice as many drops, because each dose must be activated with equal drops of either 50% citric acid drops or 4% HCl drops.*

| MMS1 Capsule Size and Dosage ||
Capsule Size	Total Drops
Size 4: holds a 3 drop dose	total 6 drops
Size 3: holds a 4 drop dose	total 8 drops
Size 2: holds a 5 drop dose	total 10 drops
Size 1: holds a 6 drop dose	total 12 drops
Size 0: holds a 7 drop dose	total 14 drops

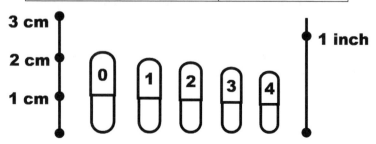

> *Note that as the capsule number gets smaller, the capsules actually are larger in size. If possible, use a capsule size that is closest to the dose size you are going to take. You can use a #0 size capsule (the large size) to take any size dose, but many people cannot easily swallow #0 capsules. Using the size capsule that corresponds with the amount of drops in your dose is best.*

> *If you have trouble swallowing capsules or pills then this method is probably not a good idea for you. Also not suggested for young children.*

Simply Can't Take One More Drop

Here I would like to address a scenario when someone feels they just can't take one more drop of MMS. Maybe they have been on a protocol for some time and they reach a point where they are not feeling all that great (this is likely because a wave of toxins are being released in the body and causing a sick feeling). Or, maybe they were not taking any MMS1, but they fall sick for one reason or another, and feel so sick that they just don't feel like they can stomach MMS1.

There is an important process at play here that I have observed over the past 22 years, and that is, that one's body can develop a revulsion to the MMS that goes far beyond bad taste. I've seen it time and time again. I believe that it is created by the pathogens. Think of it as a type a survival mechanism that protects the disease. When the disease senses that something the person is eating or taking might destroy it, the disease itself will put out a signal that creates a revulsion within the person to the substance that is going to affect it (in this case, MMS1). This revulsion can kick in when the person so much as even thinks about taking MMS1. When this happens, what can they do?

If you are sick in bed and feeling pretty bad, or if the situation develops while you are taking MMS1 and you reach a point where you can no longer stomach the idea of taking one more drop—the following procedure can be of help.

The principle here is that you do not want to stop taking MMS1 all together. Even what seems like a very, very small amount of MMS1 taken on an hourly basis can work to help rid the body of pathogens and recover health. In order to "handle" MMS1, for a period of time, you may have to reduce your dose to less than 1 drop an hour. Some have had to reduce their intake to 1/2 drop, 1/4 drop, 1/8 drop, and in extreme cases to 1/16 drop an hour. The idea is—do not quit! Even a tiny bit of MMS on an hourly basis can help your body overcome the problem.

Instructions

Step 1

❑ Please refer to the Starting Procedure (see page 79) for instructions on how to prepare a 1/4-drop dose. Once you have prepared a 1/4-drop dose you can take 1/2 of it to make a 1/8-drop dose. Or take 1/4 of the 1/4-drop dose to make a 1/16-drop dose. Prepare and take whatever small dose you have chosen for several hours, or a day or two.

Step 2

❑ Once you are comfortably taking the small amount, start slowly increasing the hourly dose. Increase slowly at a pace you are comfortable with.

❑ Keep increasing slowly, or stay low. Some people will be able to get up to a 1/4-drop dose, and then continue to increase their dosing steadily. But there are some who for various reasons cannot increase their intake of MMS beyond a fairly small amount, yet they are able to get well with low dosing. This is explained more thoroughly in Chapter 5, Health Recovery Plan (HRP) and Chapter 6, The Key Protocols.

Note: *If you have not been on a protocol and have not been taking DMSO already, but you have newly fallen sick enough to be in bed and you're feeling pretty down, do not try to use DMSO with MMS1 at this point, unless you have already been using DMSO in a protocol you are doing. (When you are feeling so sick you don't want to take anything, it's best to stick to trying to take one thing at a time. DMSO added to the MMS1 you're making an effort to take as is, might add to the difficulty. Try to build up your stamina to taking MMS1 first, before adding in DMSO.) Do not try to use DMSO when you are taking less than 1-drop doses.*

Storing MMS

The best way to store MMS (22.4% sodium chlorite in water) is in amber or green glass bottles, with a tight plastic (not metal) lid, and in a refrigerator. This is the ideal, but it isn't always possible. If amber or green glass bottles are not available, a clear bottle will do, but try to keep it out of the light (a refrigerator is dark when closed). A cool dark place will suffice if refrigerator space is not available. If glass bottles are not available, plastic bottles with plastic lids will do, but try to find bottles with a number 1 or 2 inside of a triangle on the bottom of the bottle. This signifies a better quality plastic. (Plastic classi-fied with #3 in the triangle is not recommended.) Use bottles with plastic lids as sodium chlorite (and chlorine dioxide as well) will eventually dissolve a metal lid.

Feeling Sick

If nausea, vomiting, diarrhea, or excessive tiredness occurs while taking MMS1, (see Herxheimer reaction on page 6) immediately **reduce the dose by one half but do not stop taking MMS1** unless the symptoms are too much to handle. In this case, stop altogether until the condition has cleared. Once the symptoms have cleared, then start back at one half the amount you were taking before the symptoms occurred. If you reduce the amount by one half and the above mentioned reactions continue, reduce by another half. Reduce your MMS1 intake in increments until you find the amount you can take without causing sickness from the MMS1. Even a very small amount of MMS1 on an hourly basis will help you, so the idea is to try not to quit all together if possible. When you find a comfortable amount of MMS1 that you can tolerate, stick with that for one to two days and then try to increase your intake slowly until you reach the proper amount for the protocol you are on.

Note: *If using 50% citric acid and you experience ill feelings, try 4% HCl instead. Some people cannot tolerate citric acid.*

Pregnant Women and MMS

Thousands of pregnant women have used MMS1 to restore their health when needed. Dosing for a pregnant woman is exactly the same as when not pregnant. Follow the protocols and determine what dosage is best for you. MMS1 when taken according to the protocols in this book does not harm the body and can therefore be considered safe for all people, including pregnant women, children, and babies. (Follow the proper dosages for children and babies as listed in this book—see Chapter 13.) Everyone is responsible for making their own health decisions. Check with an educated health professional, if desired.

Eating While On MMS Protocols

MMS1 doses should not be taken at mealtimes. While on the protocols, it is best to plan your meals around your dosing. Space out the MMS1 dose and meals by 20 to 30 minutes from the time you take your dose. For example, if you take your MMS1 dose at 8:00 am, breakfast could be at 8:20-8:30 am, and your next dose at 9:00 am. Your breakfast should be relatively simple and small and take no longer than 10-15 minutes to eat. Likewise if you take an MMS1 dose at 12 noon, lunch could be at 12:30 pm and so on.

During the hours you are on the protocol, it is best to try and eat smaller meals and/or snacks, as opposed to very large meals. (Don't get me wrong, you can eat while taking MMS1, just avoid the larger meals during the hours you are taking your doses.) There are a variety of ways this can be done—adjust according to your daily routine. For example, if you start your protocol fairly early in the morning, say at 8:00 am, eight hours later would be 3:00 pm, which would be the time of your last dose. If you have had smaller meals or snacks during this eight hour dosing period, and you finish your last dose at 3:00 pm, this means that by 5:00 pm or later, you could have your larger meal of the day.

Some people prefer to start their dosing later in the day, so that they are free in the morning hours to drink orange juice, or their cup of coffee or tea (see page 56 for more info). If a person starts their dosing at 3:00 pm for example, their last dose would be at 10:00 pm if on the eight hour protocol. This means that before 1:00 pm they can have their coffee, tea or orange juice—things which are not compatible with MMS1 and MMS2—at least two hours before starting the protocol. The idea is to adjust your dosing to fit your needs and schedule. See what works for you.

The effectiveness of MMS can be cancelled out when mixed with certain foods which are *particularly high* in antioxidants. I have not had the time or the resources to do a completely thorough study of all foods on the planet to see what actually *cancels out* MMS. Even if I did, there are many factors that may weigh into the equation of whether a certain food is cancelling out the effectiveness of MMS. Such as if the food is GMO, what pesticides are present, what types of additives are in the food, that might have bearing, etc. If you are very sick with a life threatening disease, to be absolutely sure if something in your diet is cancelling out MMS or not, I can suggest using the test strips (see page 278) to test compatibility of MMS with everything you eat. This may or may not be feasible for you.

Let me say, that just because a food is labeled as being antioxidant, it might not be *particularly high* in antioxidants, and thus it is not a given that it will necessarily cancel out MMS. We will continue to try and do more testing on a wide range of foods to see what is compatible with MMS and what is not. However, people have been taking MMS for 22 years and recovering their health without having so many details defined. This book gives you some guidelines on what to avoid when taking MMS. Do not take foods or supplements that are particularly high in antioxidants. Beyond that, take note of what is working or not working for you. If you don't seem to be getting results with MMS after a reasonable time on the protocol, take a serious look at your diet and see if something can be eliminated that you may suspect is conflicting with MMS. If you are accustomed to eating many items at one meal, consider going with a menu that has less ingredients. Following a mono diet (or at least a partial mono diet) during the time you are on the protocol may be a help.

To Summarize

- Do not take an MMS dose with your meals, space out food consumption and your MMS1 dose by 20-30 minutes.

- During the hours you are actually taking your MMS doses, try not to eat big "feast" types of meals, but rather eat smaller meals and/or snacks.

- Do not eat or drink things that neutralize MMS during your dosing hours. (See pages 42-45, 56.)

- If you don't seem to be having success after a reasonable time, consider simplifying your diet. Try eliminating things that could be suspect of canceling out MMS.

Nutritional Supplements and the HRP

There are two basic reasons for doing the HRP (Health Recovery Plan—see Chapter 5):

1. To eradicate a disease and recover your health.

2. For cleansing purposes, to detox and thus get rid of poisons in the body, which can then help clear up a number of health problems both small and large.

If you have a disease of most any kind then the decision is simple. What you want to do is eliminate the disease.

When someone is sick, and especially if they are seriously sick, it is a good time for the person to stop and examine various things, such as their diet and lifestyle. Eating right, exercising right, and living right all contribute to good health. While good nutrition is important for the body to get well, when someone is on the protocols described in this book, it can actually be helpful to *avoid* taking nutritional supplements for a time. This is because pathogens also feed on good nutrition, so in a sense, if you are taking nutritional supplements while the pathogens are still alive, you are building up with one hand and tearing down with the other. In addition, some nutritional supplements neutralize MMS.

This is especially true with cancer, and a number of major diseases—when you begin the protocols it is not the time to simultaneously be building up with an increase of extra nutritional supplements. In these cases, I would suggest that it is best to forgo taking supplements for two to three weeks, and possibly up to several weeks, depending on the situation. Because as I said, cancer cells and other pathogens can feed off good nutrition. You don't want to do anything to encourage cancer or other diseases to live longer or multiply. The idea is to starve and kill the disease, not give it more to thrive on.

If you have a major disease, as mentioned above, suspend or do not start any supplements as you begin taking MMS—try to give it time to sufficiently destroy the pathogens before adding in supplements. On the other hand, if you really feel the need for some type of supplements that you know are good, or you have already tried, you may want to add them in *at some point* (as suggested above, I would say not before two to three weeks for major diseases) and see how you do. It is imperative to **pay close attention to how your body is reacting.** If you are feeling good and doing better with the addition of a supplement(s), then continue. Do not change as long as you are improving. But if you do add supplements, (even though you take them at a different time than your MMS doses), and you are not progressing and getting well, or your healing is moving along too slowly, then it may be best to suspend the supplements again for a period of time.

If taking supplements, it is very important to **space them out** from the times you are taking your MMS doses by at least two hours, or even more if you can. Never take supplements at the same time you take your MMS dose.

There are just about as many nutritional theories today as there are people. But our observations indicate that it is best to use MMS to kill the cancer cells and diseases while not promoting any special nutritional boosts for the body for a time. Then, once the disease is eliminated or greatly reduced, one can build up the immune system through good nutrition. It is a step-by-step process. Detox first, before introducing any new nutritional supplements and foods.

If you do not have a major disease but just want to cleanse from various toxins and heavy metals, and elimi-nate other things such as skin problems, achy joints, various nagging irritations, and a myriad of other ailments that are not necessarily life threatening, then you may want to consider supplementation any time after the first week or two on the protocol if you believe that the supplements will be of benefit to you. But the same principles apply, if you don't feel you are getting sufficient benefit from your MMS protocol, try suspending the sup-plements for a period of time and see how you do.

Anytime you are taking vitamins and supplements while dosing with MMS, always be sure to separate the times you take these from the times you take your MMS doses, by at least two hours. If possible, take your MMS doses in the first part of the day. Then when you have completed your protocol for the day, two hours after your last MMS dose, begin taking your vitamins and supplements. It goes without saying, that if you start taking vitamins and supplements, do avoid synthetic and artificial products. It's always best to try and eat nutritious whole foods.

Food and Drink to Avoid When on an MMS Protocol

- When taking MMS1 or MMS2 avoid alcohol, chocolate, coffee, decaffeinated coffee, caffeinated drinks, tea (black, green and many herbal teas) milk, coconut water, orange juice, tangerine juice or any drinks with added Vitamin C (ascorbic acid).

- Do not take foods or supplements that are particularly high in antioxidants such as moringa, as these things cancel out the effectiveness of MMS. This is not to say you cannot have any of these foods if you are taking MMS. However when on a particular protocol it is better to wait until you finish your MMS doses for the day before consuming the above items, or take them first thing in the morning, then wait two hours before starting MMS dosing. Space them out by at least two hours after your last daily dose, or two hours before starting your daily dosing.

- If you are battling with a major disease you may want to suspend supplements all together for a time, as explained in the section above on Nutritional Supplements and the HRP.

Note: *While tea is on this list of "don'ts" there are some (not all) herbal teas that are compatible with MMS1. Use the test strip method described on page 278 to be sure what is and is not compatible.*

Chapter 4

DMSO (Dimethyl Sulfoxide)

DMSO (Dimethyl Sulfoxide), is a gentle but powerful healing substance. It is a well-known carrier solvent used widely since 1955, by alternative practitioners and a few medical doctors, as a way to carry medications deeper into the tissues and organs of the body. Taken orally, it has been used to dissolve blood clots. Body organs that are used for transplants are submersed in 99.9% DMSO to transport them between hospitals, so DMSO will not hurt tissue.

Some of the protocols in this book call for using DMSO in combination with MMS1. (Please note, you never take DMSO and MMS2 at the same time. See page 27.) This has proven to bring good results as DMSO helps to carry MMS1 deeper into tissues. DMSO by itself is also capable of relieving pain, diminishing swelling, reducing inflamma-tion, encouraging healing, antifungal, dissolving blood clots, restoring normal function of the body and much more. DMSO is often used by veterinarians and athletic coaches in the treatment of muscle sprains and various injuries. It promotes healing by increasing the blood supply to the area of the injury.

I keep some DMSO on hand at all times for use should an accident occur. It can bring amazingly quick relief to sprains and bruises, and restore the injured area in a matter of minutes if applied soon after the accident. In major accidents it can help relieve pain and help the body heal quicker than normal. The sooner it is applied after the accident the better, but if you are unable to apply it soon after an accident, it nevertheless will speed the healing process, even if there is a delay in using it. Apply DMSO directly on the injury. You can apply it full strength. If it burns or causes excessive itching add a small amount of water, a teaspoon or so, and gently rub it in. Keep adding water in small amounts if necessary, until there is no discomfort from the DMSO.

Below you will find some helpful information and things you must know about DMSO before using it as per the protocols in this book. In addition, I encourage you to research it out on the internet, where a wide range of information is available on the use of DMSO.

DMSO—Where and What to Buy

DMSO is available through various stores including animal supply companies, and online retailers such as Amazon. You want to look for the percentage (%) of "purity" on the bottle. If the bottle has "99% or 99.99% "purity or "pure" on the bottle and no other numbers, it is the highest purity.

If possible, purchase full strength DMSO (that is 99% to 99.99% purity). You can always dilute it down a little bit with distilled water if needed. If you do buy DMSO that is diluted, **purchase one that is only diluted with water**. It is sometimes diluted with *Aloe vera*, and often it is scented. I do not recommend using those. Read the labels and product description carefully. If necessary, check with your supplier to be sure what you are purchasing.

Notes

➤   *One might think that undiluted DMSO is quite strong, but keep in mind that for the most part, our protocols call* *for mixing DMSO with water. If you take it in an oral dose, you are drinking it in 1/2 cup (4 oz/120 ml) of water. If you are using it in the Patch Protocol, water is also added, so these protocols provide for diluting it. Many people can apply undiluted DMSO directly to the skin (rubbing it on, or using a spray bottle) and they do fine. If one finds this too strong however, dilute your DMSO down a bit with distilled water. It is best to start with adding a **small** amount of water, as you can always add more if needed.*

➤ *If your DMSO has been diluted with more than 10% distilled water, you can add one extra drop of that DMSO for each drop of MMS1 that is used in the protocol. For example, if the protocol calls for 3 drops of DMSO per 1 drop of MMS1, then use 4 drops of DMSO per drop of MMS1.*

➤ *It is well known that DMSO has somewhat of an unpleasant smell and taste, however, the pharmaceutical grade DMSO has been described as having **almost** no smell or bad taste. It can be found on the internet and in some pharmacies. The cost is substantially higher.*

DMSO—Allergy Test

Very, very few people, usually those with weak livers, are allergic to DMSO. To check whether or not you are allergic perform this test:

❑ Use plain water (do not use soap) and wash and dry a spot on your arm. (Just above or below the elbow works well.)

❑ Add 1 drop of DMSO (with a clean finger) to the spot on your arm and rub it in.

❑ Give the DMSO about 15 minutes to soak in and allow the area to dry.

If there is no pain in your liver area within 24 hours, it is probably safe for you to use DMSO, which will be the case for 999 out of 1000 people.

Since MMS1 heals the liver, if you have already been taking MMS1 for more than a week your liver will probably tolerate DMSO with no problem.

If you do experience pain in the liver after applying DMSO, I suggest you work on improving the condition of your liver by doing the Starting Procedure and then Protocol 1000. If you are already on a protocol, but still have a bad reaction to DMSO, simply continue with the protocol and after a few days repeat the same test again and it should show tolerance to DMSO. If you fail the test a second time, continue with the protocol and try the test every couple of days until you pass it. There has never been a report of DMSO doing any kind of permanent damage to a human since it was discovered.

DMSO—Safety Precautions

➤ DMSO is a solvent, and easily passes through the skin and into the tissues. It will also carry other substances along with it, so be careful what you have on the skin before handling DMSO.

➤ If applying DMSO topically, be sure your hands and nails are clean and free from contaminants (including soap residue) when handling DMSO. You want to also be sure the area to which you *apply* DMSO is clean.

➤ When washing an area of the skin *before* applying DMSO, it is best, if possible, to use natural, chemical-free soap to wash application areas and hands. Whether this is available or not, be sure any soap is *completely* rinsed off—or use no soap at all. Simply wash well (rubbing the skin) with clean water.

➤ The best method to apply DMSO to the skin is simply to use clean dry bare hands when rubbing the DMSO into your body or on someone else.

➤ If using bare hands to apply DMSO, do not wear finger nail polish. DMSO is a solvent that will not only dissolve the polish, but will also carry its toxic ingredients through the skin and into the body. You can cover your hand in a plastic sandwich bag (this type of plastic in general, is OK for use with DMSO) to apply the DMSO.

➤ After handling DMSO, *never wash it off with soap* as it can carry the soap into the skin/tissues. Simply rinse the hands well with clean water.

➤ Keep full strength DMSO out of your eyes.

➤ Do not use most common gloves (rubber, latex, etc.) with DMSO. It can dissolve the gloves. Even dissolving a tiny bit of the gloves can then transfer the rubber or latex into your body. Gloves made of non-stretchable plastic are OK to use with DMSO. Normally DMSO will not hurt one's hands, and gloves are not needed. (If applying frequently or in large amounts for some skin types it may cause the skin to become wrinkly, but this soon passes.)

➤ **Never add DMSO to an enema solution**. The colon contains many toxins the body is flushing out. If you put DMSO in the colon, you can return some of those toxins back into the blood stream.

WARNING

- Do not allow DMSO to come into contact with calcium hypochlorite (MMS2). This will cause immediate combustion with extreme heat and fire. In this case, it does not need a spark to start the fire instantly. Use water to put out such a fire but stand back as the water will spatter.

INGESTION WARNING

- Never use DMSO in a drink while at the same time taking calcium hypochlorite (MMS2) capsules. The DMSO can cause the MMS2 to heat and it could become very uncomfortable in your stomach. (If this should happen by accident, drink plenty of cold water to alleviate any discomfort.)

- If adding DMSO to an MMS1 dose, as per Protocol 1000 Plus for example, you must calculate no more than 3 drops of DMSO to each drop of MMS1, and it must be mixed with at least 1/2 cup (4 ounces/120 ml) of water.

- If on a protocol that calls for taking MMS2 in the same day as MMS1/DMSO doses, you can do this, but the MMS2 capsule must be separated out by one-half hour from the MMS1/DMSO doses. **Never take a dose containing DMSO and an MMS2 capsule at the same time!**

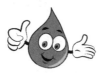

Grandson's Wart: My 8 year old grandson came to visit one weekend and had a horrible and huge wart on his knee. I actually mixed up three drops of MMS and citric acid and applied directly to the wart without diluting it at all. It did burn him a little but the next time I saw my grandson, about a month later, the wart had completely gone. It has been about a year ago now, and he has a scar where the wart was but no sign of another wart. —Tina, United States

Chapter 5

Health Recovery Plan (HRP)

Background

Good health in today's world can be difficult to achieve due to our toxic environment. Many people have complex or multiple health issues and overcoming them may require some work. For this reason I have developed this Health Recovery Plan (HRP). I sometimes think of it as the *Master Miracle Protocol*, and because it is a combination of various protocols, it truly is a Health Recovery Plan (as restoring health is a process). The good news is this: If you will follow the basic fundamentals as outlined in our Health Recovery Plan, after working with thousands of suffering people, I am confident that you will get well in a relatively short time, as others have done. Remember, MMS does not heal the body as such, it destroys pathogens and oxidizes poisons that prevent the body from healing itself. **Use this plan, as given in this book, for all diseases.**

How it Works

This book is chock full of a number of protocols that when followed properly, help restore people's health. Our Key Protocols go together with a number of Supporting Protocols to make up the Health Recovery Plan.

It is important to know that there is an overall sequence or strategy to the Health Recovery Plan. I have put it here, towards the front of this book, for an overview and for easy reference. For those who have not yet worked with MMS, at this point it may not yet make total sense how this plan works, but it will become clear as you learn the protocols outlined in this book.

The important point is that **there is a sequence of how to use the protocols.** If one's recovery comes to a standstill after the herein stated period of time, keep in mind this is always an indication it's time to change something, go to the next step, and refer often to this section of the book as needed.

All the protocols in this book can be used for children. They must, however, be adapted according to the child's weight. See Chapter 13 for instructions on how to adjust protocol dosages for children.

Overview of Key Protocols for the Health Recovery Plan

The Starting Procedure is essential to get each person started out on the right foot in an easy manner. This protocol calls for very small doses of MMS1 per hour in order to get the body accustomed to it.

Protocol 1000 is our primary protocol that kills disease pathogens, destroys poisons, and removes heavy metals from the body. We have found that a very wide range of illnesses have been overcome with Protocol 1000 alone.

Protocol 1000 Plus is a procedure that calls for the addition of a specified amount of DMSO to the dosing. The DMSO carries the MMS deeper into the tissues of the body to find and eliminate poisons and pathogens hidden there.

Protocol 2000 finishes off or does what Protocol 1000 and 1000 Plus could not do. This is our *hard hitter* that handles diseases that are so well established that they cannot be reached by Protocols 1000 and 1000 Plus alone. This is also the main protocol to overcome cancer and most life threatening diseases.

Protocol 3000 simply adds to Protocol 2000 to make it even more effective. It is an additional way of getting MMS into the body through the skin without going through the stomach as in oral doses.

The Mold/Fungus Protocol includes the addition of bentonite clay used in conjunction with MMS1. If you are not making progress with the protocols you are on, it may be necessary to switch for a time to the Mold/Fungus Protocol. You may consider starting with this protocol immediately after the Starting Procedure, but before continuing to Protocol 1000, if you feel you have come in contact with mold/fungus and suspect that mold is the root of your problem.

As mentioned above, these six protocols are our Key Protocols in the lineup for health recovery. There are a number of Supporting Protocols to go along with these depending on what the illness is. In many cases people recover their health long before they finish all of the protocols in this Health Recovery Plan. However, there are those whose illness requires going the extra mile. Some of the Supporting Protocols address specific problems and diseases and thus it is necessary to add them on (usually after Protocol 3000 but sometimes earlier) while on the Key Protocols. The instructions in this chapter will help you determine this.

Indian Herb—On rare occasions (maybe 1 out of 100) for extreme cancers, it may be necessary to use Indian Herb (or Black Salve). This herbal formula has been for sale in the United States for more than 90 years. Thousands of people have used it successfully. (See Chapter 10.)

Fundamental Principles

The simple rules with our MMS protocols and the funda-mental principles of the Health Recovery Plan, which we call the Three Golden Rules of MMS, are as follows:

➤ If you see progress—keep up with what you are doing. Do not change anything. Do not go to the next protocol. Do not increase to the next drop; when improving, just keep on doing what you have been doing until well, or until you no longer see any progress, in which case you would go to the next level.

➤ Anytime you are experiencing nausea, diarrhea, vomiting or excessive tiredness and/or are feeling worse than your illness is already making you, reduce your MMS intake by half. If these symptoms continue, then continue to reduce by one half until you are no longer feeling worse than your illness is making you feel. Then when Herxheimer symptoms (nausea, diarrhea, etc.) subside, build back up slowly to the proper dosage as per the protocol you are on, but not to the point of making yourself feel worse than your illness is already making you feel.

➤ If you do not see any progress towards healing within a five to six day period then go to the next level—ramp up—begin increasing your MMS intake. Depending where you are in following a protocol, add drops to your dose, and/or move on to the next protocol. Every time you add on a new protocol, do not stop what you are already doing. Add on, but do not stop any of the previous protocols you were following.

For example, say you are on Protocol 1000 and after the fifth or sixth day you notice some improvement in your condition, whatever it may be. The signs of improvement are an indicator to keep on with Protocol 1000, do not change anything, keep at it. On the other hand, if you are on Protocol 1000 and you have completed five or six days of the protocol and you have not noticed **any** signs of progress or improvement, then move on to Protocol 1000 Plus and so on.

Line-up of Protocols for the Health Recovery Plan

Starting Procedure: Always begin with the Starting Procedure. Simultaneously, along with the Starting Procedure, get started with the Two Fundamental Steps which are brushing your teeth with MMS1 and using the spray bottle if any skin problems exist. (Complete instructions are given on pages 73-78.) In addition, if there are any external tumors on the body, this is the time when one would also begin applying the MMS1/DMSO Patch (page 135).

Protocol 1000: Move on to Protocol 1000, and continue with this protocol as long as you see some type of improvement. But when there is a period of five or six days on Protocol 1000 and you do not see **any** signs of improvement, the first thing to do would be to make sure that the MMS is not being neutralized by anything (see pages 42-45, 52, 56). In addition, check the list for other reasons you may not be having success with MMS (Chapter 8). Then, if you are following everything correctly and you see no signs of improvement after five or six days, then go to the next level—which is Protocol 1000 Plus.

Protocol 1000 Plus: Continue on Protocol 1000 Plus as long as there is improvement, but again, if there is no improvement for a period of five or six days, once more go to the next level, which is Protocol 2000.

Protocol 2000: When on Protocol 2000, including taking MMS2 beginning on the third or fourth day, as long as you are improving continue with this protocol. But if there are no obvious signs of improvement for a period of five or six days, add on Protocol 3000.

Protocol 3000: After adding Protocol 3000, continue as long as there is improvement, but if there is a period of five or six days and no improvement, you can begin with the various Supporting Protocols. These protocols (explained further on in this book) offer additional ways to help your body recover. You keep adding on more protocols until well.

Mold/Fungus Protocol: Last, but definitely not least of Key Protocols in the line-up, is the Mold/Fungus Protocol. If you are not seeing success with Protocols 1000 through 3000, please consider switching to the Mold/Fungus Protocol for a time. There are many illnesses caused by molds/fungus so please carefully read the details explained in the Mold/Fungus Protocol on page 99.

Mold is a type of fungus. I have learned over the years, that there are some types of fungus that MMS1 and MMS2 do not seem to kill. However, I have found that when this is the case, usually clay will handle the problem. So if one is not getting the desired results with MMS1 or MMS2, it could be an indicator that mold/fungus is causing the illness and this would be a signal to add clay to your protocol.

Another important point is that I believe, as do some doctors and health practitioners, that some varieties of mold/fungus can act as a type of protective shield for some diseases in the body. When this is the case, some pathogens may not be overcome by MMS because the mold that is present provides a certain amount of "protection" for them. In this case if we eradicate the mold first with clay, as the other pathogens lose their "mold protection", MMS is then able to destroy them as well.

This may happen with both Lyme and *Candida* and possibly other diseases. *Candida* itself is a fungus and the clay can help eliminate it. But if other types of fungus are also acting as a protective shield for the *Candida,* then it is important to handle this problem first, so MMS can do its job. You can put on hold any protocol you are doing and do the Mold/Fungus Protocol anytime that you feel you need to do so. Interjecting the Mold/Fungus Protocol will not be a problem and will not harm the progress that you have already achieved, and then once you have finished the Mold/Fungus Protocol, you can go back to whatever protocol you were on and continue with it until full health is recovered.

Notes

➤   *If when taking MMS1 orally you experience burning as it goes down, or a heartburn type of sensation, this could be an indication that mold/fungus is present internally. This would be a signal to do the Mold/Fungus Protocol (see page 99). When using MMS1 externally and it burns and stings badly, use the clay and Vaseline salve (see pages 106-107).*

➤   *As has already been stated, anytime MMS makes you feel worse, (in other words, you are experiencing symptoms of a Herxheimer reaction—nausea, diarrhea, etc.) reduce the dosage by 50% but do not stop. Continue to reduce your dosage if you continue to feel worse than your illness is already making you feel. If you feel extremely bad, stop for a few hours, or a day, until the unpleasant symptoms pass, but once the symptoms do pass, start to slowly build back up your MMS intake to the proper dosage for the protocol you are on, as long as it does not make you feel sicker than your illness is already causing you to feel.*

➤   *Remember, each time you ramp up your MMS intake and add on another protocol, do not stop doing what you are already doing. Add on, but do not take away or stop what you are already doing.*

➤   *A very important thing to remember is never stop taking MMS until you are well. When well, I suggest you work on making any necessary life style changes that will help you stay healthy and fit. This may include one or more of several things. Do your best to eliminate any source of toxic poisons constantly entering into the bloodstream, such as remove root canals and attend to any infected oral cavitations, remove mold from your home and/or office, obtain a good water supply free of harmful chemicals, etc. (See Chapter 8 Reality Check, for more ideas on things you may need to change in order to stay healthy.) Make physical activity part of your daily routine. Get proper rest. Reduce stress in your life. Cultivate good relationships with others. Embrace a daily spiritual practice. Strengthen your immune system through following a good nutritional plan. Eat real food.*

Exception to the Rule

If you have cancer or another life threatening disease, it may be necessary to move more quickly into Protocol 2000 without observing the five to six day intervals before adding on a new protocol. You can determine if it is time to move more quickly by the way things are going. If you are feeling pretty bad and again, you have a life threatening disease, you may want to go at a faster pace with the protocols, but without getting sicker than you already are from your illness. In this case, even though I just said you can move more quickly, you should nevertheless, always start out with the **Starting Procedure—do not bypass this step.**

It is important to understand that the **more advanced the disease, the slower you must go to begin with.** If you detoxify the body too quickly, it can make one very sick. Getting sick, when you are already pretty ill is not a good thing. This can further weaken the body, and in the long run slow down the overall healing process.

After completing the Starting Procedure, as you move on to Protocol 1000 and the hourly 3-drop doses, if you are not seeing improvement of any kind in two to three days (instead of the standard five to six days), and if you are not experiencing a Herxheimer reaction, then move on to Protocol 1000 Plus (which is adding DMSO to your hourly doses). Then if again, you are not seeing improvement in another two or three days, move on to Protocol 2000. Follow the instructions of Protocol 2000 and continue on with the Health Recovery Plan as outlined in this book but without making yourself sicker. (See the Three Golden Rules of MMS, pages 83-84.)

Pay close attention to how your body is responding. Each person is different; some may be able to go at this fast-track pace, on the other hand, others may need to go at a slower pace than is suggested here. We have heard of remarkable recoveries from life threatening illnesses when the person took only 1 drop of MMS1 an hour. **It is not a race to see how much MMS you can handle.** Listen to your body, and remember, it is extremely important to always follow the Three Golden Rules of MMS.

Supporting Protocols—When to Add Them

In general I have recommended that one start adding on the Supporting Protocols if you have reached Protocol 3000, and have not fully recovered health. In part, this is because working through the Health Recovery Plan is a process. Overall, the body needs some time to become accustomed to each new addition in the process. Adding too many things all at once can be overwhelming, and/or possibly cause Herxheimer reaction. I do not wish for anyone to become weary and give up, which could hinder recovery. This rule of when to add on a Supporting Protocol is not hard and fast. It is a guideline.

Some exceptions when adding Supporting Protocols: It goes without saying, any time you have a persistent cough, do the Cough Protocol. A woman with breast, cervical or uterine cancer may want to begin the Douche Protocol earlier on, even as early as while on Protocol 1000 in some cases. If she is handling MMS well and feels she can add a few douches to see if that also helps her improve, it may be worth the try. Someone with colon cancer may want to add enemas or colonics at some point before reaching Protocol 3000, if they feel up to it. Another example of adding on a Supporting Protocol before reaching Protocol 3000 would be in the case of using the MMS1/DMSO Patch for any external tumors. Pay close attention to the signals of your body and follow what you feel you can handle. See Chapter 7 for a list of diseases giving you examples of using the Supporting Protocols, and when to add them into your health recovery routine.

A Word on the Additional Protocols

The Additional Protocols in this book are different than Supporting Protocols in that they are *specific* to a particular disease. Certain diseases require a different procedure than the HRP. For example, malaria requires taking two stronger than usual doses of MMS1. In most cases this eradicates malaria, but if there are complications, the Malaria Protocol gives further instructions specific to malaria.

Sometimes an Additional Protocol may suggest going to the HRP at some point, after following certain specific procedures particular to that disease. To learn more about the Additional Protocols see Chapter 11.

Two Fundamental Health Procedures for the HRP

1. Brushing Your Teeth

Almost all diseases are influenced to a large or small extent by the condition of the mouth and the teeth, therefore all protocols listed in this *MMS Health Recovery Guidebook* should be accompanied by a daily brushing of one's teeth with MMS1. It has been shown time and again that MMS1 can restore health to the mouth and in the case of doing these protocols, better results are often noticed when brushing with MMS1, even when the teeth and mouth are in very bad shape.

This does not mean that one will not need the services of a good dentist, but once the infections and diseases of the mouth are gone then the dentist can do a much better job, and the diseases of the body are 10 times more likely to be overcome. Thus a preliminary step to this recovery plan is to buy a good *soft* tooth brush for brushing teeth and gums while at the same time doing the protocols. If you use a toothbrush with toothpaste some of the time, keep a separate toothbrush that you use only with MMS1 (and DMSO if you use it). This will help avoid toothpaste residue left on the toothbrush mixing in with the MMS1. Under no circumstances should you ever use toothpaste which contains fluoride.

Brushing Teeth Procedure

Step 1

❑ In a glass activate 5 drops of MMS.

❑ After 30 seconds add only 1/4 cup (2 ounces/60 ml) of water to the MMS1 drops.

Step 2

❑ Brush both your gums and your teeth with this mixture for at least two minutes. (Pour some of the liquid over the toothbrush 3 or 4 times while brushing. See tip on page 75.)

❑ Do this 2 or 3 times a day while doing the protocols in this book.

Note: *For a number of years, people around the world have been successfully using MMS1 to keep their mouths in shape and to overcome various teeth and gum infections. You don't have to worry about the alkalinity of the sodium chlorite nor the acidity of MMS1 leaching mercury out of your teeth. This is because the acidity in the MMS activator when mixed drop for drop with the MMS (sodium chlorite) which is alkaline, is calculated to mostly cancel one another out, leaving the MMS1 solution much closer to neutral. The acidity is then much less than most fruits and cannot hurt your teeth or leach mercury from your fillings. Keep in mind that fruits and vegetables are acidic in nature more so than MMS1 doses. (For more information on the acidity and alkalinity of fruits and vegetables, see Appendix C.)*

DMSO and Teeth

If your teeth are in poor shape, for example if you have an abscess, pain, or more serious complications with your teeth, add DMSO to your teeth brushing routine. DMSO will carry the MMS right through the enamel into the tooth and can help solve many problems.

Step 1

❑ Mix up the MMS1 teeth brushing mixture described above.

❑ Brush your teeth with this mixture for a minute or so. This is for an initial cleansing of the mouth and teeth and to clear out anything you do not want DMSO to "carry" deeper into the tissues and enamel of your teeth.

❑ After this initial cleanse, rinse your mouth well.

Step 2

❑ Next, add DMSO to the rest of the MMS1 mixture and continue brushing with DMSO added. You must add DMSO to your mixture immediately before continuing to brush. Add 3 drops of DMSO for each 1 drop of MMS that you are using. For the formula above, this would be 15 drops.

❑ If you have DMSO that is already diluted some, use 4 drops for each MMS drop.

Tip: If you want to use the same solution described in the Brushing Teeth Procedure for more than one brushing, you will need to put the solution in a bottle with a tight lid. If you want to dip your toothbrush into the liquid, it is no longer reusable. So if you want to "dip" do not contaminate your entire mixture. Instead, pour part of the solution into a small glass and proceed with dipping your tooth brush into that liquid 3 or 4 times while brushing, then discard any leftover "dipping" solution. Double the amount (10 activated drops of MMS to 1/2 cup [4 ounces/120 ml] of water) to make up a portion for the day.

If you make up this solution for the day, you cannot add DMSO. **DMSO must be added immediately before use**, as over time, it will weaken your MMS solution.

2. Spraying Your Skin

While on this Health Recovery Plan, if you have *any* kind of skin problems, be it skin cancer, eczema, psoriasis, infections or wounds, etc., spraying the skin or wound with MMS is a great help. I have listed this protocol in the fundamental steps for the HRP (Health Recovery Plan), because it is important for skin problems to start right away with spraying the skin as you begin your health recovery. Using this spray bottle is also helpful for most any type of isolated skin problems as well, such as wounds or bruises, to help the overall condition of the skin, and many more conditions. It can be used for the rest of your life for skin problems, whether you are on the other protocols or not. Anytime the MMS spray stings or burns your skin go to the Mold/Fungus Protocol and check the section on the mold/fungus external procedure (see page 106).

MMS1 Spray Bottle

❑ The standard spray bottle formula is 10 to 1. That is, 10 activated drops of MMS to 1 ounce/30 ml of water.

❑ Never use tap water for any MMS mixture as it is not safe to risk getting chlorine, fluoride, or other impurities in the solution. Use only bottled drinking water, reverse osmosis, or distilled water.

❑ In most places 2 ounce or 4 ounce size spray bottles are available at the pharmacy or in health food stores.

Simply multiply the formula, 20 drops MMS1 to 2 ounces of water, or 40 drops of MMS1 to 4 ounces of water.

❑ In general this mixture will last up to a week or so. You will know that it lost its potency when the original color begins to noticeably fade.

❑ Do not leave your spray bottle in the sunlight; storing it in a dark place will help the MMS1 solution to remain strong.

❑ Use this for spraying all problems on your skin.

❑ When using an MMS1 spray bottle on your face, **avoid getting it in your eyes**.

Tip: You can spray a little on your face and then spray or pat a little DMSO (dimethyl sulfoxide, see Chapter 4) on top. Rub your face lightly to help ease wrinkles. DMSO often makes the MMS spray more effective anywhere on the body. When spraying both MMS1 or DMSO on your face, **avoid getting it in your eyes.**

Variation: If you do not see results with the 10-to-1 MMS1 spray bottle, you can increase the strength of your spray solution up to as many as 50 activated drops of MMS per 1 ounce/30 ml of water. Always begin with 10 activated drops (MMS1) per 1 ounce/30 ml, and increase the drops in increments to see what works best for you. Anytime the MMS1 spray solution stings and/or burns, regardless of how weak or strong it is, it most likely is an indication that some type of fungus is present. In this case, rinse it off with purified water and apply the clay and Vaseline salve described in the Mold/Fungus Protocol (pages 106-107).

MMS2 Spray Bottle

We have received feedback from many people who have used MMS2 in a spray bottle with positive results for the skin. Both MMS1 and MMS2 help the skin in varying ways, so try them both, and see what works best for you. Please note, in the directions below **there are some differences in the use of MMS2 and MMS1 when used in a spray bottle.**

❑ Add enough MMS2 powder (calcium hypochlorite) to a clean, dry spray bottle (a 2 ounce/60 ml or 4 ounce/120 ml size bottle works well) to just cover the bottom of the bottle.

❑ Fill the rest of the bottle with purified, distilled or reverse osmosis water.

❑ Shake it well to dissolve the MMS2 powder.

❑ Then put the MMS2 solution through a clean paper coffee filter into a clean dry glass. (If possible, use unbleached brown paper coffee filters.) MMS2 usually has small lumps that do not easily dissolve and if not strained out it will clog your spray bottle.

❑ Before putting the MMS2 solution back into the spray bottle, be sure to rinse the bottle out well with clean purified water, to be sure there are no lumps that will clog up your sprayer.

❑ When using an MMS2 spray bottle on your face, **avoid getting it in your eyes**.

Note: *Unlike the MMS1 spray bottle,* ***do not use an MMS2 spray bottle with DMSO as this could cause a burn.***

Chapter 6

The Key Protocols

Starting Procedure

This Starting Procedure must be done before following Protocols 1000, 1000 Plus, 2000 or 3000. This procedure will assure you greater success as there have been people who without it have experienced nausea, vomiting, diarrhea or excessive tiredness sometimes within the first week or so of starting Protocol 1000. Many give up right then instead of persisting. You can't blame them; they've heard how great MMS is and then it makes them feel bad, so they give up. This is because they started taking too much MMS1 too quickly to begin their protocol. Please believe me when I say that this Starting Procedure is extremely important to you for your health recovery. It can help you avoid unnecessary sickness as it helps your body gradually become accustomed to MMS.

The Starting Procedure consists of taking MMS1 in **very low doses** to start out and working up slowly to a 1-drop dose over a period of four days. (There is an exception to this rule, see variation on page 82.) MMS1 goes to work on killing the disease, but if you go too fast, the poisons from dead pathogens (any disease producing agent) builds up in the body faster than the body can get rid of them. These poisons mainly can cause nausea, vomiting, or diarrhea, and sometimes other distress, such as extreme tiredness, can also be experienced. This is called a Herxheimer reaction as explained in the definition of terms on page 6. Hopefully, going through the Starting Procedure can help one avoid or minimize a Herxheimer reaction.

Instructions for the Starting Procedure

Day One

The first day of the Starting Procedure **take 1/4 drop of activated MMS every hour for eight hours.** Since you cannot divide a drop into fourths, the following steps explain how you make the dose. Remember, use an empty, clean, dry, drinking glass. Since all MMS1 doses are taken in 1/2 cup of water, it is helpful to mark your glass at the 1/2 cup (4 ounces/120 ml) point, or use a glass with this measurement.

Step 1

❑ Activate 1 drop of MMS as per instructions in Mixing a Basic Dose of MMS1 (page 32).

Step 2

❑ Fill the glass to the 1/2 cup (4 ounces/120 ml) mark with water. Make sure the drops are mixed into the water.

Note: *Some juices and sodas are acceptable; see pages 42-45.*

Step 3

❑ Pour off 1/4 or 1 ounce/30 ml of this water mixture into another glass and drink it.

Note: Before you drink this 1 ounce/30 ml you can add a little additional water—an ounce or two at most—if you want to dilute the taste before you drink it.

❑ Discard the extra 3 ounces/90 ml. You won't be using them. **You must make up a new drink each hour;** otherwise the dose will lose its potency. Each MMS1 dose should be made up fresh—mix your drops and count to 30 seconds then add water and drink it down. One should be sure to never wait more than 60 seconds before drinking.

Day Two and Three

On the second and third day of the Starting Procedure **take 1/2 drop of MMS1 every hour for eight hours** a day.

Step 4

❑ Follow steps 1 and 2 (from day one above) each hour, but this time pour off 1/2 of the mixture (this will be 2 ounces/60 ml) and drink, and discard the other half. This gives you 1/2 drop.

Day Four

On the fourth day of the Starting Procedure **take 3/4 drop of MMS1 every hour for eight hours.**

Step 5

❑ Follow steps 1 and 2 (from day one above). In this case it would be easiest to discard 1 ounce/30 ml of liquid and drink the remaining 3 ounces/90 ml of liquid. In other words you are drinking 3/4 of the 1/2 cup (or 4 ounces/120 ml) mixture that you made in steps 1 and 2 and this then gives you 3/4 of a drop dose.

Step 6

❑ At the end of day four you have completed the Starting Procedure to Protocol 1000. The next day *(day five)*, you should begin Protocol 1000 as per the instructions on page 84.

Note: *In the case of a **very sick person,** start out the Starting Procedure with even less than the 1/4-drop dose which is suggested above. For an extremely sick person start with 1/8 drop every hour for eight hours (for one day), then do the Starting Procedure, followed by Protocol 1000.*

Variation–Fast Track for the Starting Procedure

For those of you who are familiar with MMS1 and have used it before, if you feel you would like to get through the Starting Procedure more quickly; this variation simply cuts the time in half. We do not, however, recommend this fast track method if it has been longer than approximately eight months since you have taken MMS. (If you are accustomed to taking a daily MMS maintenance dose [see page 200] and you want to start a full MMS protocol, I recommend that you nevertheless begin with the Starting Procedure using this fast track version.) In any case, before proceeding with this method remember, pay attention to how your body is reacting, go at your own pace and again, if nausea, vomiting or diarrhea occur, immediately reduce the dose by one half and follow the instructions regarding feeling sick on page 50. To fast track the Starting Procedure, simply cut the time for dosing in half as follows:

Day One—Fast Track

❑ Take a 1/4-drop dose for four hours instead of eight hours.

❑ At the end of four hours, increase to a 1/2-drop dose for the remaining four hours of day one.

Day Two—Fast Track

❑ Take a 1/2-drop dose for four hours.

❑ Increase the dose to a 3/4-drop dose for the remaining four hours of day two.

Day Three—Fast Track

❑ Start on Protocol 1000, beginning with a 1-drop dose. Follow the Protocol 1000 instructions.

Three Golden Rules of MMS

1. If it ain't broke, don't fix it! As long as you are getting better, don't change what you are doing—keep at it since it is obviously working.

2. Your body knows best...You just have to learn to listen to it! Anytime you are experiencing nausea, diarrhea, vomiting, or excessive tiredness, and/or are feeling worse than your illness is already making you, reduce your MMS intake by half and then when the sickness subsides, build back up slowly. Continuing to increase your dosage when you are feeling sicker is a common mistake. Don't let it happen to you! More is not always better. Listen to your body!

3. If you are in a rut, it's time for a change! Have you come to a stalemate? If a five to six day period passes and you do not see any signs of improvement, and you've checked to see you are not doing anything wrong, (see Reality Check, Chapter 8), go on to the next level. Depending on where you are, add another drop to your dose, do the next increase, or go to the next protocol and/or add in a Supporting Protocol as listed in the HRP. Anytime you move forward, do not stop doing what you have already been doing. Add on, but do not take away.

In Brief...
Three Golden Rules of MMS

1 Getting better? Do not change anything. Continue with what you are doing.

2 Feeling worse? Reduce your MMS intake by 50%.

3 Not getting better/not getting worse? If there are no signs of improvement, do the next increase or go to the next protocol according to the HRP.

Protocol 1000

This protocol alone has proven time and time again to restore health to people with a wide variety of diseases and conditions such as Hepatitis A, B and C, HIV/AIDS, arthritis, acid reflux, kidney disease, any number of aches and pains, urinary tract infections, depression, diabetes, and the list goes on and on. Protocol 1000 is also helpful for a good general cleanse to rid the body of unwanted toxins that one often does not even realize they have. Many people report that they really didn't feel they had any major health problems, yet after doing Protocol 1000 they felt so much better—they had more energy and vitality, clearer thinking, and felt healthier overall after completing Protocol 1000.

The instructions given here are for the original, and what I like to call, Classic Protocol 1000. If you do further research you will find that we and many other people have tried various versions of Protocol 1000 over the years. While most all of the slight variations of Protocol 1000 have been successful, according to reports we have received from around the world, the success has never been as good as the original protocol of mixing the dose fresh every hour.

Protocol 1000 is taking a maximum of 3 drops of activated MMS (MMS1) in 4 ounces/120 ml of water (some juices are acceptable, as explained on pages 42-45) once each hour, for eight consecutive hours, every day, for three weeks or until well. One does not start out at 3 drops an hour. You try to build up to 3 drops slowly as stated in this book and abiding by the Three Golden Rules of MMS. Remember, if your body does not tolerate an increase of drops, stick with what works best for you. Your health may be recovered taking less than 3 drops in each dose. Some people have recovered their health taking 1 or 2 (or even less) drops per hour.

It is best to start out slow and build up to the 3-drop dose. **Do not start Protocol 1000 until you have completed the Starting Procedure**. After finishing the Starting Procedure we start Protocol 1000 at 1 drop an hour and work up to the suggested 3-drop dose per hour.

Instructions for Protocol 1000

Step 1

❑ In a clean, dry glass activate 1 drop of MMS as per the instructions in Mixing a Basic Dose of MMS1, page 32.

❑ Add 1/2 cup (4 ounces/120 ml) of water or other recommended mixer.

Step 2

❑ Drink down your 1-drop dose within one minute of mixing.

Step 3

❑ Continue taking a 1-drop dose every hour until you are ready to increase your drops.

Step 4

❑ If after three or four hours there is no problem of nausea or any worse feeling, then increase your dose by at least 1/2 drop. Go at your own pace, (without getting sicker than your illness is already making you) but steadily build up to a 3-drop dose every hour. For example, one person might start out the first day with a 1-drop dose for two to three hours, and then they may increase to 1-1/2 drops for a couple of hours, and then 2 drops for a couple of hours and so on. Others might want to stick to a 1-drop dose every hour for the entire first day, and then 2 drops every hour the next day and so on. Some may even find it necessary to stay at a 1-drop dose every hour for a few days before they can go up.

Step 5

❑ Continue taking 3-drop doses every hour, for eight consecutive hours a day, for 21 days. You may get well without another hitch, but if at any time you experience nausea, vomiting, diarrhea, or excessive tiredness simply reduce the amount of drops you are taking by at least one half. Remember, **reduce but do not stop.** (A little bit of loose stool or diarrhea might be considered OK and part of the cleansing process, but if it becomes too much or you are also experiencing nausea and vomiting cut back immediately. Follow the instructions in the section Feeling Sick, page 50.) Be sure to follow the Three Golden Rules of MMS.

Notes

➤ *Never go beyond a 3-drop dose each hour while on Protocol 1000.*

➤ *Though it is not pleasant to feel nausea, diarrhea, vomiting, or excessive tiredness should you experience these symptoms, it is usually a sign that your body is going through the detoxification process—so on that score it is positive. The goal, however, is to go at a steady pace, not too fast, so that you do not make yourself sick.*

➤ *In the event that you recover your health in less than three weeks, I suggest that you nevertheless continue Protocol 1000 for the entire 21 day period. This will help complete the detoxification process.*

Protocol 1000 Plus

Protocol 1000 Plus requires the addition of DMSO (dimethyl sulfoxide) to your hourly dosing. Before proceeding

with this protocol, please thoroughly read and/or familiarize yourself with Chapter 4 in this book.

This protocol is simply adding DMSO to the MMS1 Protocol
1000 dose which is 3 activated drops per hour (or sometimes less). With Protocol 1000 Plus, you add in 3 drops
of DMSO for each drop of MMS. Or, in case you have not
progressed to 3 drops an hour by this time, continue the
same amount of MMS1 you've been taking and add in the
DMSO accordingly. For example, if you are taking a
3-drop dose of MMS1, you would add 9 drops of DMSO.
If you are taking a 2-drop dose of MMS1, you would add
6 drops of DMSO.

Instructions for Protocol 1000 Plus

Step 1

❑ Activate 3 drops of MMS. (If you have not been able
to work up to a 3-drop dose yet, due to nausea, etc.,
activate however many drops you are taking.)

❑ Add 1/2 cup (4 ounces/120 ml) of water (or compatible
liquid; see pages 42-45, 56).

Step 2

❑ Immediately after adding the water, add in 3 drops of
DMSO for each drop of MMS1 you are using. For
example, if you are making a 3-drop MMS1 dose, add
9 drops of DMSO. (Thoroughly mix in the DMSO by
stirring it.)

❑ Drink down the dose immediately as once the DMSO
is added the MMS1 will begin to slowly lose potency if
left to sit.

Step 3

❑ If after adding DMSO to your dose you experience discomfort (such as nausea, diarrhea, etc.), reduce the amount of DMSO you are adding on the next dose. Instead of adding 3 drops of DMSO per 1 drop of MMS1, reduce to 2 drops of DMSO to 1 drop of MMS1. If you still have discomfort, reduce the DMSO by another drop, in other words, use 1 drop of DMSO per 1 drop of MMS1. If you still experience discomfort after reducing the amount of DMSO 2 times, then completely stop adding DMSO to your MMS1 doses for a day. Then start back with small doses of DMSO and build up slowly to 3 drops of DMSO per 1 drop of MMS1.

Notes

➤ *An important reason to drink the MMS1/DMSO dose immediately is because DMSO begins to cause the dose to slowly lose its potency. It takes up to six hours to lose full potency; nevertheless, it is best to drink it straight away so it doesn't lose any of its power. I suggest drinking it within one minute of adding DMSO drops, because it loses a large amount of potency in the first ten minutes and then continues to lose potency at a slower pace.*

➤ *When progressing from Protocol 1000 Plus to Protocol 2000, always continue using DMSO according to the instructions given here in Protocol 1000 Plus while doing Protocol 2000, i.e. always add 3 drops of DMSO to the dose for every 1 drop of MMS1.*

Protocol 2000

Protocol 2000 is, in essence, our Cancer Protocol, but we are not naming it "Cancer Protocol" as such because it also works well for most other life-threatening diseases. I have observed that more than 90% of those who use Protocol 2000 faithfully, and take responsibility for using it as directed here, overcome their cancer or other disease completely. However, I must also mention that there are cases of cancer and other diseases that simply are too far gone for even MMS1 and MMS2 to help. Normally these are the cases that have had tremendous amounts of chemo, radiation, or surgery treatment and the body is simply "past the point of no return." However, we never say never. If the person still has one more hour to live, get some MMS1 into him. See page 249 for more information on helping people with extreme conditions.

On Protocol 2000 you will:

- Increase the number of drops you take each hour to as many drops as you can handle (up to the maximum amount of drops for your weight—see page 92) without getting sick due to the MMS. In most cases the increase in drops is needed for cancer and other life-threatening diseases.

- Increase the number of hours you take your dose each day from eight to ten hours.

- At the beginning of the third or fourth day of Protocol 2000, you should begin taking MMS2 in addition to MMS1.

The most important thing to remember is, **never stop taking MMS until you are well**. Remain on Protocol 2000 and any needed Supporting Protocols, as explained in the Health Recovery Plan, until you have fully recovered your health.

Note: *When progressing from Protocol 1000 Plus to Protocol 2000, always continue using DMSO according to the instructions given in Protocol 1000 Plus while doing*

Protocol 2000, i.e. add 3 drops of DMSO to the dose for every 1 drop of MMS1.

Instructions for Protocol 2000

Step 1

❑ Increase the number of hours per day that one takes the hourly dose to ten hours per day instead of the eight hours per day of Protocol 1000.

Step 2

❑ Begin increasing the drops in your daily dose by 1 drop increments. For example, if you were taking 3 drops an hour as per Protocol 1000, you can increase to 4 drops.

❑ The Health Recovery Plan (HRP) gives allowance for an exception to the rule, (see page 70). If you fall into this category and therefore come to Protocol 2000 directly from the Starting Procedure because of cancer or some other life-threatening disease, then begin at 1 drop per hour and increase the drops per hour after only a few hours at 1 drop per hour. You can tell if you should not add another drop per hour by the way you feel. Just keep increasing by 1 additional drop per hour until a tiny sickish feeling beyond how the disease makes you feel, lets you know for the time being to stop increasing. Some people can move along quicker and some cannot, please be attentive to the Three Golden Rules of MMS.

❑ It is important to not allow yourself to feel worse than your disease is already making you feel, as the additional sickness can then slow your recovery down. So if taking your MMS dose results in nausea, vomiting, diarrhea or excessive tiredness reduce the number of drops you are taking by 50% for the next dose, if it still seems like the MMS1 is continuing to cause distress, then decrease the dose by another 50% of what you are taking. When you feel comfortable with the amount of MMS1 you are taking, then slowly increase the drops again. If the added sickness is severe then temporarily stop taking the drops altogether and start again as soon as you are feeling better. And again, increase to as much as you can take without feeling worse than you already are.

The following chart gives the theoretical maximum amount of drops that most people should take for their body weight. Anyone weighing more than 200 pounds can calculate their maximum number of drops by adding 1 drop for each 20 pounds over 200 pounds. There are times when a cancer is not improving that one might go ahead and take more drops per hour than suggested here, in that case do not hesitate to do so, but normally this chart is correct. Remember, follow the Three Golden Rules of MMS. Some people will not get up to anywhere near these amounts. These are maximum amounts—they are not a goal.

Protocol 2000 —Maximum MMS1 Dosage	
Weight	Dosage
80-100 lbs (36-45 kg)	Take no more than 8 drops hourly
100-120 lbs (45-54 kg)	Take no more than 8 drops hourly
120-140 lbs (54-63 kg)	Take no more than 9 drops hourly
140-160 lbs (63-72 kg)	Take no more than 10 drops hourly
160-180 lbs (72-81 kg)	Take no more than 11 drops hourly
180-200 lbs (81-90 kg)	Take no more than 12 drops hourly
200 lbs (90 kg) and above: Increase the maximum dose by 1 drop for each additional 20 lbs (9 kg)	

Step 3

❑ Begin taking MMS2 on the third or fourth day into the protocol. (Please read section MMS2—Details, page 274, for information on where to purchase calcium hypochlorite, and instructions on how to make MMS2 capsules.)

❑ Use either #1 size capsules which are the smallest that you should use, or #0 size capsules, which is one size larger than #1. (And no, I didn't make a mistake on capsule sizes; they really get smaller in size as you increase the number.) Start by loading the #1 size capsules 1/8 full or #0 size capsule about 1/16 full. When the capsules are pulled apart, one side is always larger than the other side. Fill the larger side (pack loosely). Then put the smaller side on and be sure you push it down securely in place.

Step 4

❑ Step 3 gets you started, but increase the amount you put in the capsule **over the next several days,** working up to either full for #1 size capsule, or 3/4 full for a #0 size capsule. Slowly increase the amount you put in the capsule.

Step 5

❑ Take one of these capsules 5 times a day—once every two hours.

❑ Take your first MMS2 capsule one-half hour after taking your second MMS1 dose of the day.

Sample Time Schedule for Protocol 2000, Once MMS2 is Added to Your Dosing

Protocol 2000 MMS2 Time Schedule	
Time	**Dose**
9:00 AM	MMS1 dose
10:00 AM	MMS1 dose
10:30 AM	MMS2 dose
11:00 AM	MMS1 dose
12:00 PM	MMS1 dose
12:30 PM	MMS2 dose
1:00 PM	MMS1 dose
2:00 PM	MMS1 dose
2:30 PM	MMS2 dose
3:00 PM	MMS1 dose
4:00 PM	MMS1 dose
4:30 PM	MMS2 dose
5:00 PM	MMS1 dose
6:00 PM	MMS1 dose
6:30 PM	MMS2 dose

Notes

➤ *While working up to the correct size capsules of MMS2, which is either a full #1 size capsule, or a 3/4 full #0 size capsule **(never go beyond these amounts)**, keep your MMS1 doses constant. In other words, do not be working on increasing your drops of MMS1, while you are working up to your proper dose of MMS2, because if you get nauseous you will not be able to determine which of the two might be causing you to feel sick. Once you have reached the suggested amount of MMS2, then you can begin increasing your drops of MMS1 once more.*

➤ *Remember, at any time, whether you are increasing your amounts of MMS1, or MMS2, if at any time you feel nauseous or sick from the increase, decrease the amount by at least one half and build back up slowly.*

➤ **Never take a dose containing DMSO and an MMS2 capsule at the same time!** *See pages 23-24 for the full warning on this.*

Protocol 3000

The goal with serious or life-threatening situations is to quickly get MMS1 circulating in the blood while trying to stay under the nausea level. One way to achieve this is by using DMSO with MMS1 topically. DMSO is a carrier and therefore takes MMS1 directly into the skin and tissues and thus into the blood. Testing under laboratory conditions by adding tiny non-dangerous amounts of radiation have demonstrated that DMSO carries MMS1 directly to any cancer in the body and it then penetrates the cancer cells. We have evidence that DMSO also carries MMS1 to any place in the body where disease has weakened the area. (For further information I recommend Stanley Jacob's book: *Dimethyl Sulfoxide (DMSO) in Trauma and Disease* by Stanley W. Jacob and Jack C. De La Torre. Also *The DMSO Handbook* by Hartmut P.A. Fischer.)

Protocol 3000 is the topical use of MMS1 mixed with DMSO, applied to the body every hour for a minimum of eight hours a day. The MMS1/DMSO procedure described below is an accelerated skin technique that helps push MMS1 into the blood plasma. This method also helps to avoid a Herxheimer reaction. In the case of cancer or other life-threatening disease, it should be used in addition to a normal oral regimen of Protocol 2000.

Instructions for Protocol 3000

Step 1

❏ Mix up a solution of 10 drops of MMS with 10 drops of 50% citric acid or 10 drops of 4% HCl acid. Count 30 seconds for activation.

❏ Add 20 drops of water. But if this mixture is too strong (causes burning of the skin or other irritation), add more drops of water until it doesn't cause irritation. If there is no extra skin sensitivity, you may want to add *less* water (do this in increments), to see if you can tolerate a stronger mixture.

❏ Add 1 teaspoon/5 ml of DMSO.

❏ Immediately spread the mixture over one arm. You can use your hand to spread the mix. (Be sure your hands are washed and thoroughly rinsed so as to remove all of the soap **before** applying DMSO.) It is not necessary, and even potentially dangerous to wear a glove, (if latex or rubber). When you have finished, wash your hand with plain water, do not wash with soap and water, as DMSO is a carrier and can carry some of the soap into your tissues.

Step 2

❏ The following hour, mix up another MMS1/DMSO solution and spread it on your other arm. Repeat the next hour and do a different part of your body. Do one arm first, then the other arm, then a leg, then the other leg, then your stomach, and then back to the first arm, and so on. Use a different part of the body each time you apply the DMSO/MMS1 combination. Do this once every hour for eight consecutive hours.

Step 3

❑ Repeat this process once every hour for eight consecutive hours for three consecutive days. (It is fine to bathe or shower after completing the hours applying the MMS1/DMSO. Wait at least one hour after applying the last application. Thoroughly rinse well with plain water before using soap.)

Step 4

❑ Then take a break. Quit from one to four days or however many days it takes to overcome any problems that may be caused by the DMSO (such as extra dry skin).

Step 5

❑ After the first week you can use this topical application four days a week, or more, if there is no problem with your skin. If there is no problem, continue to use MMS1 and DMSO every day, as long as there is no skin irritation. Anytime you experience irritation, cut back for a time, or you can add more water to the mixture.

Note: *When you quit the MMS1/DMSO topical application for four days you should still continue with your other MMS protocols.*

Variations

➤ An alternative method is using the same mixture as mentioned above of MMS1 drops to water, but spread this mixture on the body first and then spray DMSO (see pages 261-264 on DMSO spray bottle), or pat on the DMSO over the top of the MMS1 on the same area. Gently rub it into the skin. You can use your clean bare hands to do this.

When finished rinse your hands with plain water. (Remember, DMSO is a carrier, so using it with soap could carry the soap into your system, so rinse with water and wipe dry.)

➤ For extra sick people who should take smaller doses of DMSO, it would be best to start out using only a small area of the body. I suggest using an area about the size of the palm of your hand—no larger. Use a small area like this for several days before going to a larger area such as the entire arm or leg. Use a larger area only if there is no adverse reaction to DMSO in the smaller area.

➤ Or instead, add extra water to the mixture. That is, instead of using a smaller area to rub the DMSO on, add extra water to the MMS1/DMSO solution and then put it on the entire arm or leg and other areas.

➤ There is a more convenient way to do this protocol that involves using spray bottles to apply the MMS1 and DMSO to the body. You can find the full details of the spray bottle method for Protocol 3000, in the section for children in this book on page 260. The same procedure and mixture for children can be used for adults. Although the spray bottle method may be easier for some people, I have left the original method for this protocol above for the sake of learning, and for the sake of those people who, for one reason or another, may not be able to obtain spray bottles.

Cautions

➤ When working with DMSO, do not use rubber or latex gloves or other medical gloves. You could get rubber into your body as DMSO melts the rubber. The plastic gloves that are not stretch are one kind of plastic that can be used with DMSO.

➤ Keep full strength DMSO out of your eyes. Be careful not to touch your eyes when handling DMSO until you have rinsed the DMSO off of your hands.

➤ If you notice a burning sensation on your skin after you have applied DMSO, a good technique is to place a teaspoon of purified water on the burning area and gently rub it in. Keep adding water until it is no longer burning. Or use a spray bottle with plain water in it for such problems, but do rub the water in.

➤ You can rub olive oil or *Aloe vera* gel on the skin after the DMSO/MMS1 application in order to soothe the skin if you feel burning or irritation.

Note: *For a complete list of safety precautions for overall use of DMSO please see pages 25-27.*

Mold/Fungus Protocol

Mold can be a contributing factor to many illnesses. Mold can make its way into some surprising places. While many of us associate mold with damp or humid climates, the truth is, mold can be found almost anywhere, even in dry climates. The trouble with mold is that it can often be difficult to detect. When one is sick due to mold, it can affect the body in a variety of ways, and the symptoms can vary greatly. Mold can cause infections; it can wreak havoc in the respiratory track, causing all types of lung problems, difficulty breathing, coughing and wheezing. It can cause a variety of skin problems, headaches, depression, memory loss, visual problems, allergies, sinus and nasal problems, muscle and joint pains, digestive disorders, immune system disturbances, fatigue, and much more. Needless to say, mold can be the culprit in making people terribly sick.

Under some conditions mold/fungus can spread throughout your body quickly. Sometimes it will make you sick,
and other times you may not feel it for days or months. It
might even come and go without you ever feeling it.
However, don't bet on that, as it can also hang on for
months or even years, ruining your health and making
you susceptible to many other diseases.

Mold is a type of fungus. I have learned over the years,
that there are some types of fungus that MMS1 and MMS2
do not seem to kill. Why? I'm not exactly sure. But I have
found that when this is the case, usually clay will handle
the problem. So if one is not getting the desired results
with MMS, it could be an indicator that mold/fungus is
causing the illness and this would be a signal to add clay
to your protocol. I have personally had success doing this,
as have many others. I'm not going to guarantee it will
work for you, but in my opinion, if someone is experiencing one or many of the symptoms described above and is
not having success with MMS, it is certainly worth a try to
add clay to your protocol and see if it brings results. Clay
should not hurt you or slow your progress. Millions of
people have been ingesting clay for hundreds of years.

**Some indications that mold/fungus is at the root of
illness, and the kind(s) MMS will not help include:**

- If the problem is external and MMS is sprayed on
  the fungus, it will become painful and start to sting
  and burn badly.

- If the fungus is in the mouth when MMS1 is applied,
  the mouth will sting and burn. (Rinse your mouth
  out with cool water to get rid of the sting caused
  by the MMS.)

- If mold is a problem internally, and while taking
  MMS orally you experience burning as it goes down,

or a heartburn type of sensation, this could indicate mold/fungus is present internally.

If the above reactions occur, this Mold/Fungus Protocol, with the addition of clay, may remedy the situation. Clay has millions of tiny holes with a powerful electrical charge in each hole. Microorganisms are pulled into the hole by the attraction of the charge and are trapped in the hole. The clay then washes out of the body taking the microorganisms with it (either alive or dead). The procedure given below has proven to be successful with many people.

The clay I recommend to use for this protocol has several names: Aztec clay, bentonite clay (calcium bentonite is preferred), or montmorillonite clay (from France).

Instructions for Internal Use of Clay

If you have not been on an MMS protocol, do the Starting Procedure (page 79) first, before beginning this Mold/Fungus Protocol. After completing the Starting Procedure in four days, go right into this protocol on the fifth day. If you are already on an MMS protocol and determine you need to stop for some days to do the Mold/Fungus Protocol, when adding clay into your MMS routine—for a short period of time—while doing Steps 1 and 2 of this protocol, **discontinue** taking your MMS doses as per whatever protocol you may be doing at the time (Protocols 1000, 1000 Plus, 2000 or 3000).

Step 1

❏ On day one of taking clay, take 5 doses of clay, each dose two hours apart.

❏ **Clay dose 1 and 2:** Add 1/2 level teaspoon (2.5 ml) of clay in 1/2 cup (4 ounces/120 ml) of water. It is best to continue stirring the water as you sprinkle the clay into the water. Drink it down. It is OK to drink slowly but keep it stirred.

❑ **Clay doses 3, 4, and 5**: Add 1 level teaspoon (5 ml) of clay in 1/2 cup (4 ounces/120 ml) of water. Stir as mentioned above until it is thoroughly mixed with the water. Drink it down. It is OK to drink slowly but keep it stirred since clay will quickly settle back down to the bottom of the glass.

Step 2

❑ If after the first day of taking the clay you are feeling OK and experience no extra sick feeling (no sicker than you were already feeling with your sickness) after 5 doses of clay, proceed to Step 3 below on day two. However, if it seems like you are feeling a little bit worse than normal, continue drinking the clay doses described in Step 1 above, for one more day, taking a clay dose every two hours until you have taken 5 doses, then proceed to Step 3 on the third day.

Step 3

❑ Alternate the clay drink described in Step 1 above with whatever your MMS1 dosage was before starting the clay. (The first hour take an MMS1 dose, the next hour take a clay dose, the next hour an MMS1 dose, the next hour a clay dose and so on.) For example, if you have begun doing this Mold/Fungus Protocol just after finishing the Starting Procedure, then start with 1-drop doses for this step. If you were on Protocol 1000 taking a 3-drop dose of MMS1 every hour, alternate that dosage with your clay dose. Or, if you were on Protocol 2000 taking a 5-drop dose of MMS1 every hour, alternate that dosage with your clay dose. Alternate each hour for eight hours. This would be 4 doses of MMS1 and 4 doses of clay each day.

❑ Do the alternating doses for two days. If you are on this step and you are seeing improvement, keep it up (as long as there is improvement of some kind) until you are completely well. But, if you reach a point where you go several days without any type of improvement go to Step 4 below.

Additional Important Information for Step 3

➤ If you were on Protocol 1000 Plus and adding DMSO to your MMS1 doses at the time you started taking clay, you can also continue adding DMSO to your MMS1 doses while doing Step 3 above.

➤ If you were on Protocol 2000, however, **do not continue with MMS2 during the time you are taking clay and MMS1** as per Step 3 above—simply continue with the amount of MMS1 you were taking at the time you started the clay, be it 5-drop doses, 7-drop doses, etc.

Step 4

In this step you will take the clay and MMS1 in the same dose. When mixing clay in an MMS1 dose, I suggest using fizzy mineral water (carbonated water). This is because the carbonation in fizzy mineral water tends to protect and preserve MMS1 as it is mixed with the clay. The clay tends to minimize the strength of MMS1 over time, but by mixing it with fizzy water, it will not minimize it as quickly.

To further explain why taking clay mixed with MMS1 may be beneficial: Mold almost always suppresses your immune system thus allowing other pathogens to take hold. I believe in this case, the other pathogens may not be overcome by MMS1 because when mold is present it provides a certain amount of "protection" for them. Thus if we eradicate the mold with clay, as the other pathogens lose their "mold protection" MMS1 is then able to destroy them as well.

❑ In a clean dry glass activate your MMS drops, using the same amount of drops you were taking in Step 3.

❑ Immediately add 2 ounces/60 ml of fizzy mineral water (carbonated water), followed by 1 level teaspoon of clay. I find it helps to "sprinkle" the clay into the glass while stirring the liquid. It will foam up a bit, don't let that startle you, just be sure to have a big enough glass so it does not overflow.

❑ Once the clay is sprinkled in and completely mixed then you can add another 2 ounces/60 ml of the carbonated water.

❑ Drink this dose **slowly** if possible, over a period of five minutes.

❑ Do this every hour, for a total of eight hours for at least one day.

Notes

➤ *The clay tends to mask the taste of MMS1, however, if taste is still an issue for you, you can use a soft drink such as Pepsi, Coke, Sprite, etc., as per the guidelines on pages 42-45 in this book. (Do not use orange soda.) My prefer-ence if possible, is the fizzy mineral water, as it does not contain sugar.*

➤ *You can make this same drink with purified bottled water that has no carbonation, it will still help, but it will not be as potent as when done with carbonated water or soda.*

Step 5

❑ If Step 4 is making you feel better and you feel you are improving, continue more days as long as you are improving, but once you stop improving, (or if you feel you are well) stop taking the MMS1/clay doses. If you have an internal mold/fungus problem, the clay added to your protocol should help knock it out. Normally it is not needed to continue this step for a prolonged period of time, usually a few days does it, but be sure to continue for as long as you see improvement.

Notes

➤ *If you are living or working in a location with a lot of mold, you should continue taking the clay at least with a maintenance dose of 6 drops of MMS1 and 1/2 level teaspoon of clay until you have eradicated the mold problem in your home or workplace.*

➤ *Once you are well you can then continue with daily MMS1 maintenance doses (see page 200). On the other hand, if you have stopped seeing improvement and thus stopped the MMS1/clay doses but you still feel sick, it may be a good idea to go back to whatever protocol you were on, (taking the amount of MMS1 and/or MMS2 you were taking before adding the clay), for another period of time. This would be to further clean out any pathogens or toxins that the clay helped to trap that still need to be flushed out of the body, or those the mold/fungus may have been "protecting". It may be that there are some remnants of poisons and pathogens that are still present even though the mold is gone, thus one should continue with the former protocol until you are sure you are well.*

➤ *If you are experiencing mucous in the throat and/or coughing, I suggest you drink your clay doses slowly over a couple minutes, giving the clay time to work in the mouth, throat and esophagus as it goes down. It's also a good idea to swish it around in the mouth a few times before swallowing.*

➤ *When taking clay internally, be sure your bowels are moving so you can eliminate the toxins which the clay is pulling out. In the case of constipation, I have found the herb, Senna, to be one of the best solutions. It is natural and it exercises the colon. Senna can be found in tablet form (sold as a laxative) in health food stores and in some countries in pharmacies. Start out with the recommended dose and increase the number of tablets every four hours until you have success.*

➤ *We have explained above that if MMS1 or MMS2 seem to not be helping an illness, it may be due to mold/fungus. There are however, other reasons why one may not be having success with MMS, please review Chapter 8.*

Mold/Fungus External Procedure

There are many types of fungus that can manifest externally on the body. As mentioned earlier, one indicator that MMS1 will not be helpful occurs when MMS1 is sprayed on or otherwise applied to the fungus. It will become painful and start to sting and burn badly. In this case, the MMS1 will actually make the condition worse, and it's best to try another course of action, such as given below.

Instructions for Mold/Fungus External Procedure

Step 1

❑ Mix well equal parts of clay with Vaseline Petroleum Jelly. Alternatives to Petroleum Jelly are coconut oil, olive oil, or another good quality carrier oil. Make the mixture fairly stiff so that it will adhere well to the fungus area.

Step 2

❑ Smear this salve on the fungus and cover with a gauze bandage.

❑ If the fungus is on your feet, smear the clay mixture on the feet, put on clean socks and put your shoes on if needed.

Step 3

❑ Every four hours, wash the area and then apply more of the mixture until the fungus is gone.

Notes

➤ *Depending on how sensitive the area of skin is, it can be painful to wash off a Vaseline mixture. We have found the Vaseline with the clay mixed in tends to soak into skin after some hours. Use a very mild soap, if possible one made with natural ingredients (those free of perfumes are best, as perfume can tend to irritate tender and damaged skin) and warm water. Pour the water slowly over the area and massage it very gently with your hand. Gently pat dry with a clean towel or gauze pad.*

➤ *There are various brands of Petroleum Jelly on the market. I recommend the "Vaseline" brand (the original, which is triple-purified to be 100% pure) for mixing with clay to make a salve. Vaseline has the unique ability to wet and penetrate and remain in place on the skin for hours longer than most oils. Sometimes coconut oil, olive oil and other oils can be used to carry various medicinal substances to the skin and hold them there. However, nothing matches the ability of Vaseline to hold healing substances in contact with skin for hours, while at the same time acting as a healing agent itself. Use the various other oils only if you cannot obtain Vaseline.*

An Important Review

The HRP and the Key Protocols offer various options. You have the exception to the rule (page 70), where if needed you can move more quickly into Protocol 2000. There is a fast track option (page 82) for the Starting Procedure. In Protocol 2000, you'll find maximum dosage amounts. All of this would seem to point to the more MMS one takes the better. This is *not* necessarily so!

Always remember, it is *imperative* to follow the Three Golden Rules of MMS. Your own body will tell you what your personal ideal dose is. Most people will never get up to anywhere near the maximum dosage amounts. These are *maximum* amounts—they are not a goal. Such amounts may be needed for some, but not for others.

You may be able to take a certain amount of MMS, say a 3-drop dose for Protocol 1000, for one illness. But then down the road sometime if you need to repeat the proto- col, you may find you can only handle 1 drop an hour, even though last year you did 3 drops an hour with no problem. Why is this? Our bodies change; different types of pathogens or toxins, or different amounts of pathogens or toxins may contribute to varied reactions. Any number of circumstances and conditions may have bearing on how much MMS you can tolerate. This is why it is so important to pay attention to the signals your body is giving you, and why I want to repeat, it is not a race to see how much MMS you can take.

Each person is different, for some people a fast track approach or higher dosing may be needed, and for others, low dosing brings results. As I have mentioned earlier, we have had some people with advanced cancers get well on only 1-drop doses of MMS each hour and low doses of MMS2, and some on even less, a 1/4 or 1/2 drop dose.

Chapter 7

HRP and Various Diseases

Using the HRP in Conjunction with Supporting Protocols for Various Diseases

In this book it is not possible to list all of the diseases of mankind, nor even all of the illnesses and conditions that we know from feedback, that MMS has helped. However, below I have listed some of the more common diseases to show a general idea of how we use the Health Recovery Plan (Chapter 5). This plan refers to using the Key Protocols in conjunction with the Supporting Protocols, the Additional Protocols and sometimes Indian Herb when needed.

It is important to note that in order to incorporate the suggestions below into your personal health recovery routine, you must have a good understanding of the Health Recovery Plan and how it works. Remember, the HRP begins with the Starting Procedure, and then one follows the proper sequence of the Key Protocols in accordance with the Three Golden Rules of MMS (see pages 83-84). Depending on the illness/disease, other Supporting Protocols and/or Additional Protocols are also added in if needed.

I have emphasized in the Health Recovery Plan to always begin with the Starting Procedure (see page 79), and then proceed to Protocol 1000. However, there are some diseases which I believe it would be beneficial after completing the Starting Procedure, to first do the Mold/Fungus Protocol, and then proceed to Protocol 1000 and continue with the rest of the HRP as outlined in Chapter 5. This is because mold and fungus are often a big part of the problem. In the list below I have noted which diseases would be beneficial to go to the Mold/Fungus Protocol after completing the Starting Procedure, and before doing Protocol 1000. However, **any time there is a question as to what you should do or what you should start with, always begin with the Starting Procedure and follow the standard HRP.** Any time that you feel that you are not making sufficient progress during your HRP program, you can always switch to the Mold/Fungus Protocol for a certain time period.

Aches and Pains: Do Protocol 6 and 6. Then go on to the Starting Procedure and continue following the HRP. Simultaneously, while on the Starting Procedure use the MMS1 spray bottle, along with DMSO. Spray MMS1 on the pain area followed by DMSO (either spray DMSO on, or rub it on by hand) 4 or 5 times a day. Continue with the HRP until the pains are gone. Always follow the Three Golden Rules of MMS.

Acid Reflux: Begin with the Starting Procedure. Then go on to the Mold/Fungus Protocol, first, before continuing on to Protocol 1000 and following the HRP as needed (always observing the Three Golden Rules). Take a good brand of probiotics at any meal that is separate by at least two hours from your MMS doses, for at least a month. Continue until well.

Allergies: Begin with the Starting Procedure and continue following the HRP (always observing the Three Golden Rules) until allergies are gone.

Appendicitis: If one so chooses, do Protocol 6 and 6 (page 169). If there is still pain an hour after taking the second 6-drop dose, one may need to go to the hospital. However, if the pain is mostly gone, in this case skip to Protocol 1000 and start with taking a 3–drop dose of MMS1 every hour. Since the appendix is connected to the digestive system this will keep a flow of MMS1 going directly to the appendix and help it heal. Pay careful attention to the Three Golden Rules of MMS. If feeling better, continue with Protocol 1000 for three weeks in order to detox the system. If pain returns, it may be necessary to go to the hospital.

Arthritis: Begin the HRP. Simultaneously, while on the Starting Procedure use the MMS1 spray bottle, along with DMSO. Spray MMS1 on the pain area followed by DMSO (either spray DMSO on, or rub it on by hand) 4 or 5 times a day. Continue following the HRP plan through the Key Protocols, as needed. Arthritis comes in many different degrees of intensity. The problem may be remedied by following the Starting Procedure and Protocol 1000, or it may necessitate following through with the full procedure of adding in all the various Supporting Protocols as out-lined in the Diseases Generally Considered Incurable section (see page 117). Remember to follow the Three Golden Rules. Continue until well.

Asthma: Begin with the Starting Procedure. Then go on to the Mold/Fungus Protocol, first, before continuing on to Protocol 1000 and following the HRP as needed (always observing the Three Golden Rules) until well.

Autoimmune Diseases: Autoimmune disease affects millions and millions of people worldwide. There are as many as 80 types of autoimmune diseases (and count-ing). Some of the more common ones range from lupus, to celiac spruce disease, to inflammatory bowel diseases, to psoriasis, and the list continues. MMS has been known to remedy these and many others. Begin with the Starting Procedure and continue following the HRP (always observing the Three Golden Rules). Many autoimmune diseases have similar symptoms, which makes them very difficult to diagnose. It's also possible to have more than one at the same time. If at any time during your HRP program you are not seeing sufficient progress, it may be helpful to stop and do the Mold/Fungus Protocol and see if that helps. With some autoimmune diseases it may also be necessary to add on Supporting Protocols if needed as suggested in the Diseases Generally Considered Incurable section (see page 117).

Candida: Begin with the Starting Procedure. Then go on to the Mold/Fungus Protocol, first, before continuing on to Protocol 1000 and following the HRP as needed (always observing the Three Golden Rules) until well. Simultaneously enemas and/or colonics (see pages 148-153) can be added in whenever one feels ready, usually do not start until you have started Protocol 1000.

Common Cold: When you feel a cold coming on, do Protocol 6 and 6. If the cold is gone one hour after the second 6-drop dose, that is all that is needed for a cold. If the cold persists after doing Protocol 6 and 6, begin the Starting Procedure and continue following the HRP (always observing the Three Golden Rules) until well. It is important to note that the body sometimes uses the common cold to detoxify. When this is the case, no amount of MMS or any medication will quickly stop a cold—it will simply need to run its course. In this case, do not stop taking MMS as with MMS the cold will usually clear up much sooner than normal—even if it's the type of cold that the body uses for detoxification, which may take two or three weeks to completely overcome.

COPD (Chronic Obstructive Pulmonary Disease): Begin with the Starting Procedure. Then go on to the

Mold/Fungus Protocol, first, before continuing on to Protocol 1000 and following the HRP as needed (always observing the Three Golden Rules). When finished with the Mold/Fungus Protocol, simultaneously as you begin Protocol 1000, start the Lung Protocol (the Cup) see page 159.

Crohn's Disease: Begin with the Starting Procedure and continue following the HRP (always observing the Three Golden Rules). Enemas, and if possible some colonics, can help. In the case of this particular disease, get started on the enemas or colonics as soon as you are accustomed to doing the protocols. It is best to start with an enema or two to see how it goes (see page 148). If you notice improvement, continue as long as you are doing better. Do not do enemas or colonics for Crohn's disease without including MMS1 drops. If the first enema goes well, you can increase the number of MMS1 drops in the next few enemas according to the instructions. If doing colonics, follow the instructions on page 152. Keep in mind a colonic is really a super enema and it does clean the colon more efficiently. Remember the Three Golden Rules of MMS still apply, especially if you are getting better, don't change anything.

Dengue Fever: Follow the protocol for dengue fever on page 190.

Dental Issues: Do the Brushing Teeth Procedure (see page 73). Simultaneously, begin with the Starting Procedure and continue following the HRP (always observing the Three Golden Rules).

Depression: Begin with the Starting Procedure and continue following the HRP (always observing the Three Golden Rules) until well. If needed, continue with the program for Diseases Generally Considered Incurable section (see page 117).

Diabetes (Type 1 and 2): Begin with the Starting Procedure and continue following the HRP (always observing the Three Golden Rules) until well.

Digestive Problems: Begin with the Starting Procedure and continue following the HRP (always observing the Three Golden Rules) until well. In addition, take a good probiotic with meals eaten two hours apart from MMS doses, which means two hours before starting MMS dosing and two hours after the last dose of the day, for at least a month.

Ear Infections: Immediately do the Ear Protocol (see pages 139-141). Simultaneously, begin with the Starting Procedure and, if needed, continue following the HRP (always observing the Three Golden Rules) until well.

Eczema: Begin spraying the affected area with the MMS1 spray bottle (page 76) and apply DMSO on top. At the same time begin the Starting Procedure and continue following the HRP (always observing the Three Golden Rules). If the MMS1 spray burns and stings it is an indication that mold/fungus may be present. In that case follow the instructions in the Mold/Fungus Protocol (see page 99) for overcoming mold and fungus on the skin. Continue following the HRP until well.

Erectile Dysfunction: Begin with the Starting Procedure and continue following the HRP (always observing the Three Golden Rules) until well.

Eye Disease: Immediately do the Eye Protocol (see page 137). Simultaneously, begin with the Starting Procedure and continue following the HRP (always observing the Three Golden Rules) until well.

Fibromyalgia: Begin with the Starting Procedure and continue following the HRP (always observing the Three Golden Rules) until well.

Hepatitis A, B, C: Begin with the Starting Procedure and continue following the HRP (always observing the Three Golden Rules) until well.

Herpes (all types): Begin with the Starting Procedure. Then go on to the Mold/Fungus Protocol, first, before continuing on to Protocol 1000 and following the HRP as needed (always observing the Three Golden Rules) until well.

High Blood Pressure: Begin with the Starting Procedure and continue following the HRP (always observing the Three Golden Rules) until well.

HIV/AIDS: Begin with the Starting Procedure and continue following the HRP (always observing the Three Golden Rules) until well.

Infectious Diseases: These can be caused both by viruses or bacteria, and both can be inside the body and on the skin. Pneumonia, meningitis and diarrhea, for example, can be caused by either viruses or bacteria. In addition, there are thousands of skin diseases caused by viruses and bacteria, examples are chicken pox rashes, roseola, and shingles. Antibacterial drugs can sometimes stop bacterial [infections] diseases but medicine has yet to develop anything to stop viral infections. Thankfully, MMS has been known to stop both viral and bacterial diseases. **For either viral or bacterial infections,** begin with the Starting Procedure and continue following the HRP (always observing the Three Golden Rules) until well. In the case of viral or bacterial diseases on the skin, use the MMS1 or the MMS2 spray bottle, (see page 76). If spraying the skin causes stinging or burning, it is an indication that mold or fungus is present. In this case follow the instructions for the mold/fungus external procedure on page 106.

Kidney or Liver Disease: Begin with the Starting Procedure and continue following the HRP (always observing the Three Golden Rules) until well.

Lyme Disease: Begin with the Starting Procedure. Then go on to the Mold/Fungus Protocol, first, before continuing on to Protocol 1000 and following the HRP as needed (always observing the Three Golden Rules) until well.

Malaria: Follow the Malaria Protocol (see page 180).

MRSA: Follow the MRSA Protocol (see page 196).

Obesity: Begin with the Starting Procedure and continue following the HRP (always observing the Three Golden Rules) until well. Some changes in diet and life-style may be necessary.

Parasites: Begin with the Starting Procedure and continue following the HRP (always observing the Three Golden Rules) until well.

Prostate (high PSA): Begin with the Starting Procedure and continue following the HRP (always observing the Three Golden Rules) until well.

Sinus Problems: Do the MMS1 Nose Procedure. Simultaneously, begin with the Starting Procedure and, if needed, continue following the HRP (always observing the Three Golden Rules) until well.

Skin Problems: Begin with the Starting Procedure and continue following the HRP (always observing the Three Golden Rules). Use an MMS spray bottle, and spray the affected area up to 5 times a day. Add DMSO immediately on top of the spray and gently rub it in. (Only add DMSO on top of the spray if it is MMS1. **Do not use DMSO with an MMS2** spray bottle, see page 78.)

Tumors and Cysts: Begin with the Starting Procedure and continue following the HRP (always observing the Three Golden Rules). If the tumor or cyst is on the outside of the body use an MMS spray bottle on it 5 times a day including using DMSO each time. (**Do not use DMSO if you are using an MMS2 spray bottle,** see page 78.) The MMS1/DMSO Patch can also be applied to external tumors and cysts.

Urinary Tract Infections: Begin with the Starting Procedure and continue following the HRP (always observing the Three Golden Rules). In addition, for both men and women, use an eye dropper to gently inject into the urinary tract (through the opening in the head of the penis for men, and through the urinary opening [outer opening of urethra] for women), a full squeeze of the MMS1 liquid from an MMS1 spray bottle made according to the instructions for an MMS1 spray bottle (see pages 76-77). This can be done 4 or 5 times a day.

Diseases
Generally Considered Incurable

There are many diseases generally considered to be *incurable*. We have nevertheless received countless reports from people worldwide who through using MMS have been recovered to full health from many of these supposedly incurable diseases. Some of these include ALS (Lou Gehrig's Disease), Alzheimer's, autism, cancer (all kinds), leukemia, multiple sclerosis, Parkinson's, polio, rheumatoid arthritis, and many other life threatening diseases.

If you or a loved one is suffering with an incurable or life-threatening disease I suggest the following:

➤ Begin with the Starting Procedure. Then go on to the Mold/Fungus Protocol, first, before continuing on to Protocol 1000 and following the HRP as needed. Always observe the Three Golden Rules of MMS, which tell you when to go to the next step or to the next protocol. Keep moving forward all the way through Protocol 3000 if needed.

➤ If you reach Protocol 3000, and are still not completely well, then start adding on the Supporting Protocols. At this point, the idea is to try and get MMS into the body in more and varying ways. Think of it as hitting the disease from every possible angle. The idea is not to add on every single Supporting Protocol all in the same day. But try to add on more and more as you go. If you can't do some of these things at first, don't worry, just keep at it until you are doing them all. When you start adding on Supporting Protocols, keep taking MMS1 and MMS2 oral doses and applying MMS1 and DMSO externally, according to where you are in your progress with the Key Protocols. Remember, a very important principle, you add on, but do not take away what you are already doing. Always follow the Three Golden Rules of MMS.

Note: *For the most part, I suggest you add on Supporting Protocols in the order listed below. There are some exceptions to this rule, depending on your illness, on how you feel and how your body is responding. Please read Supporting Protocols—When to Add Them (page 71), for more details on this.*

Baths: Do full baths with MMS1. In a few days switch to MMS2 baths if you can. If you see the need to continue MMS baths, alternate the baths between MMS1 and MMS2—see what works best for you. (See pages 142-

148.) If full baths are not feasible, then do the foot bath. You may want to do a combination of the three different baths. Take notice of progress with the baths and follow what is working for you.

Enemas: You can also try two enemas a day. In the case of serious disease I also recommend at least two colonics a week which replaces enemas and is more far reaching than an enema (see pages 148-153).

MMS Bag Protocol: Try doing several of these a week (see page 156).

Douche Protocol: Women can also add douches into their health recovery plan (see page 153).

MMS1/DMSO Patch Protocol: Depending on what the problem is, for example in the case of external tumors, you may also want to do the MMS1/DMSO Patch during this time.

Indian Herb: If, after doing all of the protocols outlined in the Health Recovery Plan along with the Supporting Protocols, you have not recovered your health, then using Indian Herb is the next course of action (see Chapter 10).

This may seem to be a tough program. You will know if you are getting better or not. It's hard work and it takes determination, but many people have been successful at it and have overcome their particular disease and live happy, productive lives as a result.

Lyme Success: Last march I got what I thought was the flu. It was the worst flu I had ever had in my life. I hurt from every pore of my body. I began to take machinate but it didn't help. Since I had MMS in the house I decided to give it a try. Well that did the trick! I felt well again within a short time. I stopped taking it since I seemed to be back to my old self. After a couple of days, the symptoms came back and that's when I realized that I was dealing with some other illness and not the flu. It took a lot of investigative work to discover that I had Lyme disease. My medical doctor was absolutely no help at all. In fact she was a hindrance. I went online and used a symptom checker and it indicated I probably had MS or Lyme. Since the MMS was helping, I began using it again, and researched as much as I could on how to treat my symptoms. I began Protocol 2000. I also contacted a naturopathic doctor in my city for support. To my great surprise, she supported using MMS. She recommended using MMS in an enema which helped a lot. I am using MMS2 as well. Both protocols work well together. If it were not for MMS I believe I would be in the hospital fighting for my life right now. My symptoms were severe and the pain was horrible. MMS is a miracle in my opinion! —Brenda B., Canada

Throat Cancer: Treating a guy with throat cancer. His blood count is back up, gained a little weight, and his doctor said whatever he is doing to keep doing it because it is working. UPDATE: The guy with throat cancer has been completely cleared of his throat cancer. I'm so excited for him and the fact that it just makes people better.—C. P., United States

Chapter 8
Reality Check

Reasons Why You May Not Be Having Complete Success with MMS

1. Not Following the Protocol Carefully Enough: These protocols are the result of 22 years of helping people recover their health. There are reasons for the exact process given. Those who try to change the process or who are not diligent in following the procedures exactly can fail. If you are serious about wanting to be in good health, or you want to live if you have a lethal disease, please follow the protocols exactly.

It is important to note that there are many internet sites that have various protocol and dosing suggestions (using MMS) for a myriad of health problems. Many of **these sites are not accurate**, and give information which is not what we have found to be effective over the past 22 years. We simply have no control over everyone who has jumped on the MMS bandwagon and who put out incorrect information. I urge you to follow the instructions in this book, which is my most up-to-date information. If you wish to glean more information from the internet, be sure it is from a trusted site.

2. Changing the Dosing when One is Improving: Remember, when you are noticing some improvement large or small, do not change anything, but keep doing what you are doing until there is no more improvement for a five to six day period. What often happens is when someone feels he is getting better he will think, "If I'm getting better with this amount of MMS, more MMS will help me get better quicker." So even though he is improving, he ups his dose. When this happens the additional MMS1 may kill off too many pathogens at once, causing a Herxheimer reaction that could bring on headache, extreme tiredness, nausea, vomiting, and/or diarrhea. The person may become discouraged and quit taking MMS altogether. So remember, as long as you are improving, don't change anything, and only go to the next higher protocol when you have not seen any improvement for a five to six day period.

3. Neutralizing MMS in the Body: Coffee, decaffeinated coffee, caffeinated tea, some herbal teas, milk, alcohol, coconut water, orange juice, tangerine juice and all juices with added Vitamin C or ascorbic acid, will directly neutralize MMS. (Vitamin C naturally found in fruits and vegetables in moderate amounts are OK.) Foods and supplements that have exceptionally high amounts of antioxidants such as moringa, must not be taken while on the MMS protocols. (See pages 42-45, 52, 56.)

4. Pharmaceuticals: Up until this point in time, we have not noticed any reactions with MMS and medical drugs, although we cannot guarantee this will always be the case. The decision to take or not to take pharmaceutical drugs is a personal one. Medications affect each person's body in different ways. We cannot say across the board in every case that taking prescription drugs will inhibit health recovery with MMS. However, we have seen a trend that continuing to take pharmaceuticals while doing the MMS protocols will often slow health recovery, or prevent it all together. If one has made a decision to not take pharmaceuticals, occasionally they may need to continue with a pharmaceutical drug (while on the MMS protocol) for several days or a week or more (depending upon the situation and the kind and amount of medications you must wean off of). This is to prevent bad reactions from occurring in the first several days due to "drug shock" when the medications are first stopped. Usually it is best to wind down slowly by reducing the drug in steps. The right qualified alternative health professional can help you safely wean yourself off of the medications.

5. Quality and Strength of your MMS and Activator:
Sometimes one might purchase bottles of MMS that do not have the required potency (usually from an unap-proved source) and thus the drops will make a weaker dose. One way to make sure the dose is the proper strength is to make sure that the drops turn amber color after mixing MMS and activator drops and counting 30 seconds, (see page 39); if not something is wrong. If they do not turn amber but merely turn yellow, only use those drops for a few days until you get good ingredients—MMS and activator. Either one or both could be bad. If the drops do not even turn yellow, do not use them.

6. Taking Supplements while on the MMS Protocols:
Vitamins, minerals, and other supplements that one might add to the diet, should be suspended for a time while on MMS protocols. This especially includes foods with high amounts of antioxidants. MMS removes poisons and destroys bio-films that protect pathogens. It then kills the pathogens, and this aids in healing. Supplements not only aid the body, but they feed pathogens as well. Unfortunately, most of the time the pathogens are first in line to get nutrition from the supplements and thus one is furnishing nutrients to the disease while also trying to kill it. For this reason, supplements can slow down health recovery or even stop it altogether. On the other hand, after one has been on a protocol for two or three weeks, and has followed all the rules, as they continue on their MMS protocol, then they might consider taking supple-

ments if they feel the need. Remember, separate any supplements from MMS dosages by at least two hours. Follow the lead of the body and determine if the supplements are helping or possibly hindering MMS from fully working. Please read the nutritional supplement section beginning on page 53 for a full explanation.

7. Previous Therapies: We have had people come to us *on their last leg* who have had multiple chemotherapy treatments, radiation and surgeries which makes it difficult to restore health. MMS has the additional burden of removing toxic chemotherapy drugs. In this case, usually the immune system is compromised, and the removal of various organs makes the recovery a little longer or often considerably longer. Therefore, previous therapies, depending upon the amount and to what degree followed, can prolong health recovery. You may have to keep at it longer than expected.

8. Attitude Can Slow Healing: It's understandable when you are sick and feeling rotten that you may fall into complaining or being negative. However, many studies have proven that having a positive attitude and keeping complaining to a minimum contributes to faster recovery. Attitude very seldom keeps MMS from working altogether, but a poor attitude can affect the immune system, and slow down the healing process, sometimes considerably.

9. Blood Testing: There are many times when blood tests can make it look like MMS is not working. The best way to determine if MMS is working is by tangible results. How do you feel? Are you gaining or losing weight as necessary? Are sores healing and skin rashes disappearing? Is a general sense of well-being restored? If you have all these positive signs and yet a blood test shows a problem, the test is probably wrong.

With HIV/AIDS, hepatitis C, and some other diseases, often times at the first testing during and after an MMS cleanse, the blood virus count can go extremely high. This is always a good indicator that MMS is working, and the count will soon go low. What happens is MMS destroys the viruses. However, the white blood cells continue to absorb the dead or dying viruses. When this happens, the cells get more and more stuffed until they burst, releasing huge amounts of the dead/dying viruses. These dead/dying viruses are counted in the viral load, but they are all eventually cleaned out of the blood naturally by the body. When this cleaning process is complete, then the viral load will drop to zero. If someone who is using MMS does not understand this, they may believe they are not getting better and may stop using MMS.

You must leave a sufficient amount of time before blood tests will read accurately, and this depends upon the illness. Also remember, many labs make mistakes, therefore more than one opinion is often a wise choice. But most of all go by how you feel. If energy is restored and wounds disappear, you can pretty much know that you are healed, or at least that you are getting better.

10. Vaccines: It is a known fact that vaccines often contain weak pathogens of many kinds of diseases. Many of these diseases can actively affect the body. In addition to the disease, it is also a known fact that most vaccines contain mercury and other chemicals that are extremely poisonous, and in most cases, these toxins slow healing considerably. However, we have almost always seen that MMS protocols eventually overcome the poisons caused by the vaccines and health is then recovered. If you must get a vaccination while on an MMS protocol, I suggest that you follow the Vaccine Procedure on the day you receive the vaccine (see page 173) and then continue with the MMS protocol that you were on. Generally, MMS can overcome the negative effects of most or all vaccines.

11. Pressure from Family and Friends: Family and friends can discourage one from doing the protocols by being negative about what is being taken as well as doubting it will even work. This outside influence can often cause one to decide to stop taking MMS either entirely or from doing the protocols correctly.

12. Environmental Poisons: There are hundreds if not thousands of sources of poisons in our surroundings that all of us come in contact with regularly. If one is trying to restore health and is constantly in contact with toxins, the body's immune system can be occupied with trying to eliminate these toxins and healing can be slowed down or stopped altogether. In this case, one may have to remove himself from the toxic situation before full healing takes place.

13. Mold/Fungus: Mold is a type of fungus. There are some types of mold that are unaffected by MMS. They affect the inside of the body as well as the outside. Mold/fungus can enter the mouth and digestive system and do a great deal of damage to one's health, as well as create bad sores and rashes on the skin. When MMS is not effective against certain types of mold/fungus, clay can often remedy the problem. It is important to keep in mind that you can distinguish mold/fungus from other sores and pathogens by the fact that when MMS is applied, it not only stings and burns, but it can also make the condition worse. Aztec clay, also called bentonite clay, or montmorillinite clay, usually will kill the mold/fungus that MMS will not eradicate. (See page 99 for the complete Mold/Fungus Protocol, including further details on how to recognize mold in or on your body.)

14. Re-infection: Just because a person has completely restored health, does not mean that they cannot re-infect themselves again. If one continues a lifestyle or habits that caused the disease to begin with, or is continually exposed to a certain disease or toxin again after they have had their health restored, then re-infection can occur. Consider a lifestyle change and then repeat the protocol.

15. Self-deception: People can deceive themselves into thinking they are well when in fact they are still sick. One must accept reality and take personal responsibility for one's health and continue with the protocols until all symptoms are gone no matter how long it takes.

16. High Tension Wires and Microwaves: It has long been thought that those living close to high tension wires and microwave towers have a much higher incidence of cancer and disease than those who do not. At least the wires and towers are suspect. Alternative medicine prac-titioners often advise sick people to move away from locations near such wires and towers. I have been told by some people that they did feel better after moving. So if one finds that he still feels bad after doing a protocol and yet is in close range to these things, this is something to consider. Even simple changes can help, such as using wired internet instead of WiFi in the home, and using cell phones set so they work on speakerphone instead of held up to the ear.

There is a lot of controversy as to the safety or dangers of food heated or cooked in a microwave oven. If I was trying to restore my health, I personally would think twice before having a microwave in my home. If you are not making sufficient progress with your MMS protocols, and you are using a microwave oven, you may want to discontinue its use for a period of time and see if it helps. Here are some links to articles that you may find helpful in making your own decision about using a microwave oven:

The Hidden Hazards of Microwave Cooking, by Anthony Wayne and Lawrence Newell:
http://www.health
science.com/microwave_hazards.html

Mercola on Microwave Ovens:
http://articles.mercola.com/sites/articles/archive/2010/
05/18/microwave-hazards.aspx

Microwave Ovens Destroy Nutritional Value of Your Food, by Mike Adams:
http://www.naturalnews.com/021966_microwaves_mic
rowave_ovens.html

17. Chlorine and Fluoride: These two poisons are in many public water systems around the world. In locations where they haven't been allowed to dump the industrial waste called fluoride into the water, they have been able to use chlorine. Both are toxic and both are carcinogenic (cancer causing). At the very least, following an MMS protocol using water containing fluoride or chlorine can slow down the recovery process. Please consider using reverse osmosis water, distilled water, or bottled water that does not have either one of these poisons added or used in any way.

18. Oral Pathology: A substantial impediment to complete healing is oftentimes oral pathology. Deadly anaerobic bacteria routinely exist in root canals, under crowns, and even in previous extraction sites (causing decay of the jawbone called cavitations). Most of these bacteria cannot be reached by the immune system and can cause low grade infections that persist for years, eventually causing heart conditions, auto-immune diseases, arthritis and more. Many times the oral pathology causing various problems in the body can be overcome by the proper brushing with MMS1 and DMSO (see page 73), however in rare cases this will not solve the problem, and in this case consulting with a high level biological dentist may be necessary to help MMS1 completely restore health.

19. Biofilm: If a biofilm is present in the body, it can prolong or prevent healing. If one is not aware that a biofilm is present, they could think that MMS is not working or not working adequately, and give up on doing the protocol. Please see page 273 for more information on biofilm.

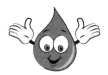

Bladder Cancer: A friend of mine went to the emergency room because he was urinating blood. After that, doctors found out that he had a bladder cancer. He was sent home. Then doctors wanted to start chemotherapy, but he did not have insurance, so it took time to go back to the doctor. I gave him MMS and he started to take it every hour. He took MMS for 2 weeks. Then he stopped because he started to have a diarrhea and vomiting and he had enough of it. During that time he was qualified for insurance. He went back to the doctor to get chemotherapy, but before, the chemotherapy doctor went inside his bladder to check the size of the cancer. They were very surprised when they found out that there was no cancer. —Tadeusz, United States

৯৩

MMS Works: It is safe. I have used doses ranging from 2 to 12 drops, from one to four times per day. I am 56 years of age and have used MMS off and on for a decade. And it virtually saved my daughter's life. —Wayne F., Canada

In Brief...

Three Golden Rules of MMS

1. Getting better?

Do not change anything.
Continue with what you are doing.

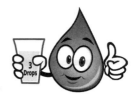

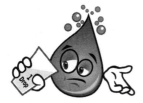

2. Feeling worse?

Reduce your MMS intake by 50%.

3. Not getting better/not getting worse?

If there are no signs of improvement,
do the next increase or go to the next
protocol according to the HRP.

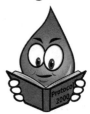

Chapter 9

Supporting Protocols

Cough Protocol

Many illnesses produce coughing and some produce extreme continuous coughing. Coughing zaps a person of energy, usually energy that is needed to help overcome the sickness. I have seen coughing continue on and on for weeks and sometimes even months.

Coughing can prevent health recovery and often can cause a sickness to worsen. One's muscles in his stomach can become extremely sore and likewise one's throat can become sore from coughing. Coughing can prevent sleep which is also debilitating. The fact is that prolonged coughing presents a major problem. The protocol below offers an alternative to taking drugs (for a persistent cough) which often have serious side effects. I have seen this work for others and myself; I believe it can work for you.

Coughing is caused by mucus and how the body reacts to it. Almost all diseases produce mucus in the area that they exist. For example, sickness in the lungs produces mucus in the lungs, and likewise sickness in the gut often produces mucus in the gut. Coughing, especially strong coughing, is the body's effort to keep the windpipe (trachea) free of mucus. Blockage of the windpipe is an extreme problem. The body cannot allow this to happen or death results, thus the body's natural reaction is deep, heavy, uncontrollable coughing in order to expel mucus from the windpipe. Even the smallest amount of it threatens to block breathing.

Mucus can vary from watery to very hard. One can cough for hours to just expel a tiny bit of mucus from some areas of the windpipe. On occasions, coughing does not stop when all of the mucus has been removed from the breathing tubes because certain types of mucus may still be present in the mouth and throat. This mucus may be caused by other pathogens not related to the original cause of the coughing. Coughing will occur as long as certain types of mucus are in the mouth or throat. This mucus can be so thin that it is watery and it will even drip out of the nose when coughing, or it can be very thick and continue to collect in the throat, and it needs to be spit out.

Thus removing all mucus from inside of the entire mouth which includes the teeth, gums, the sides of the cheeks and throat, is needed.

Once this is accomplished coughing should stop, this is almost always the case, but if coughing does not stop then you would need to repeat the steps given below a second time.

Instructions for Mucus Removal

Mucus removal from the mouth can be accomplished with the use of various acids in a diluted form. Drops from a bottle of MMS activator such as 50% citric acid or 4% hydrochloric acid (HCl), or 1/2 squeezed lemon or lime can be used.

Note: *Using acid or lemon in these dilute forms will not hurt your teeth. You can rinse your mouth with plain clean water when you have finished each session. I do not* *recommend using baking soda or alkaline water to neutral-ize the acid, rinsing with clean water is sufficient.*

Step 1

❑ Add 20 drops of either 50% citric acid or 4% HCl acid (from a bottle of MMS activator), to 1/2 cup (4 ounces/120 ml) of water. Or use 1/2 squeezed lemon or lime in 1/2 cup of water. (Twenty drops of MMS activator acid in 1/2 cup of water is a very weak acid. It is much weaker than lemon juice and is easy to use.)

❑ Add 1 drop of unactivated MMS to this solution and wait three minutes before using.

Step 2

❑ Take a sip (about 1 tablespoon) of the mixture from the 1/2 cup you made in Step 1. Swish the water around several times in your mouth making sure it thoroughly covers your teeth and the sides of your mouth. If you have false teeth make sure the water gets under the teeth as well.

❑ After swishing, tip your head back and gargle for a few seconds and then spit the water/acid mixture out.

❑ Repeat this step 1 more time.

Step 3

❑ Using a soft tooth brush, (make sure the toothbrush is clean with no toothpaste on it) pour a little of the solution that is left of the 1/2 cup (4 ounces/120 ml) of acidified water that you made in Step 1 over the toothbrush. Brush your teeth and gums for one minute. This is to make sure there is no mucus film left on your teeth.

Step 4

❑ Rinse your mouth out 1 more time, with a sip (1 tablespoon or so) from the 1/2 cup of acidified water made in Step 1.

Notes

➤ *Do these four steps anytime a coughing spell comes on. Be sure to keep up with whatever protocol you are on (if any) while doing this extra procedure for a cough.*

➤ *If coughing persists, I recommend doing the Mold/Fungus Protocol (see page 99) as I have come to believe, like many other professionals, that mold can protect various diseases including diseases that create mucus that cause coughing.*

➤ *After you have completed the Mold/Fungus Protocol, if coughing is still a problem, then I suggest the following: Start over again with the Starting Procedure and work through the Health Recovery Plan. Whether prior to doing the Cough Protocol you were already on an MMS protocol such as Protocol 1000 or 2000, or if you were not on any MMS protocol, whatever the case may be—go to the Starting Procedure. Simultaneously, at this point please review Chapter 8 and carefully consider if something stands in the way of your health recovery. Anytime you are on an MMS protocol, as a rule, coughing should stop. This is why I suggest you review what might be hindering your recovery, correct anything that may be wrong, and start over from the beginning.*

MMS1/DMSO Patch Protocol

The MMS1 patch is another way to use MMS1 and DMSO topically. This is not the same as Protocol 3000 per se, but it is a variation of how to use MMS1/DMSO externally in an effective way to heal all types of skin issues. We have had success with many types of tumors, cancer tumors, and infections such as MRSA, diabetic ulcers, and other skin diseases. It has brought relief to pain areas especially when cancer is present. While Protocol 3000 is one way to absorb chlorine dioxide into the body, through the skin, the patch is designed to target a specific area of the skin.

Note: *See page 265 for instructions on preparing an MMS1/DMSO patch for a child.*

Instructions for MMS1/DMSO Patch

Step 1

❑ Apply to clean skin. In a clean bowl activate 10 drops of MMS with 10 drops of 50% citric acid or 4% HCl. Count 30 seconds for activation.

❑ Immediately add 10 drops of purified water.

❑ Then add 10 drops of DMSO. Make sure this solution is mixed well.

Step 2

❑ Pour the solution onto a cotton gauze pad making sure the liquid is fully absorbed into the pad.

❑ Cover the problem area with the gauze pad and leave for seven minutes. The first time you do this patch, I suggest applying it for only seven minutes in order to test how the skin reacts. If it goes well, then the next patches can be held on for 15 minutes each time. If the skin is overly irritated, adjust the solution as described in the notes below.

❑ It is best to hold the patch in place as putting tape on the soaked gauze pad could have a reaction with the DMSO.

Step 3

❑ After the allotted time, remove the patch.

Notes

➤ *If the above steps cause any burning or irritation to the skin, add 10 more drops of water to the patch. If 10 drops of water doesn't stop the burning on the next patch, add another 10 drops of water, and keep adding more until there is no burning or irritation.*

➤ *Depending on the size of the area to be covered, this formula can be doubled or tripled, or cut in half accordingly. Apply once or twice a day until well.*

Eyes, Ears and Nose Protocols

Cleansing your eyes, ears, and nose with MMS can allow them to heal when nothing else will. MMS is very gentle on these delicate parts of the body. Follow the directions given below.

We never recommend using tap water for your MMS doses. Especially for the eyes, ears and nose, you want to be sure not to use tap water from your faucet to make up your mixture as almost all tap water in the USA, and many other countries, has fluoride and often chlorine as well. Do not allow these poisons in your eyes, ears or nose. Distilled water, if available, is the best choice for the Eyes, Ears and Nose Protocols, and secondly purified water. Avoid tap water altogether. **When making up these different formulas (which are not all the same), be sure to clearly mark all bottles** so as not to confuse what is what.

Eyes

In times past, I have used an eye formula of 1 activated drop of MMS to 1 ounce/30 ml of distilled water, and sometimes 1/2 drop of MMS1 to 1 ounce/30 ml of distilled water. Both of these solutions can work for some body types. However, this strength of MMS1 for the eyes has caused discomfort in some cases. I have since developed a new eye formula (below) and have come to find this weaker solution will accomplish the same purpose to overcome eye problems. A good rule of thumb is if the eye drops sting or burn more than just a few seconds, (a few seconds is normal) or to an uncomfortable degree, then it would be best to dilute your solution with distilled water. If you have test strips and can test your eye formula, the parts per million for the MMS1 eye solution outlined below should read between 6 and 10 ppm.

MMS1 Formula for Eyes

❏ Activate 1 drop of MMS with 1 drop of 4% HCl (preferred for the eyes), or 50% citric acid. Be sure you have waited the correct amount of time (30 seconds) and that the MMS liquid has turned amber in color.

❏ Add 4 ounces/120 ml of distilled or purified water to the 1 activated drop.

❑ Pour this solution into either a dropper bottle(s) or a spray bottle.

Notes

➤ *This is the basic formula for the eyes—1 activated drop of MMS to 4 ounces/120 ml of purified water.*

➤ *This mixture lasts about one week if it is in a bottle with a tight lid and kept in a cool dark place. So be sure to make up a fresh batch each week if needed. This is likely to be more than enough for eye drops or spray for a one week period for one person. The actual formula for the eyes should be a 1/4 activated drop to 1 ounce/30 ml of distilled water. However, because it is not possible to measure 1/4 of a drop on its own, we suggest mixing up your eye solution in this way.*

MMS1 Eye Procedure

These are our two preferred methods of applying the MMS1 mixture to eyes:

1. Spray bottle for eyes.

❑ Put the eye formula solution described above (1 activated drop of MMS to 4 ounces/120 ml of water), into a clean spray bottle.

❑ For the very best healing action, flush your eye or both eyes with this mixture. With your head tilted slightly back, eyes wide open and looking up towards the ceiling, spray each eye 4 to 8 times per application. Try to keep your eyes open when spraying, and then blink several times to aid the flushing. It may burn just a tiny bit at first, but if your mixture is correct, this will pass quickly.

❑ Do this 3 to 4 times a day for best results.

2. Dropper bottle for eyes.

❑ Use the same eye formula mixture (1 activated drop of MMS to 4 ounces/120 ml of water), added to a dropper bottle.

❑ Put 3 or 4 drops into each eye while blinking to spread it around.

❑ Do this 3 or 4 times a day.

Notes

➤ *For most eye problems, MMS clears things up in one to four days with some cases taking up to a week, but you can continue to use the eye solution if needed, until well.*

➤ *Use the same mixture and procedure for children.*

➤ *Use the eye spray bottle or eye dropper bottle 1 to 2 times a week for maintenance.*

➤ *Be diligent to clearly mark your bottles. You would not want to mix up a spray bottle for the skin, with a spray bottle for the eyes—they are two completely different solutions.*

Ears

Note: *The formula of the ratio of activated drops to water is different for ears and nose than that of the eyes.*

MMS1 Formula for Ears

❑ Activate 1 drop of MMS with 1 drop of 4% HCl, or 50% citric acid. Be sure you have waited the correct amount of time (30 seconds) and that the MMS1 liquid has turned amber in color.

❑ Add 1 ounce/30 ml of distilled or purified water to the 1 activated drop.

❑ This is the basic formula for ears—1 activated drop to 1 ounce/30 ml of purified water. The ear mixture lasts about one week when kept in a bottle with a tight lid and in a cool dark place. So be sure to make up a fresh batch each week if needed.

MMS1 Ear Procedure

Step 1

❑ Use the solution above, 1 activated drop to 1 ounce/30 ml of water. For adults, fill a standard eye dropper with 1 tight (full) squeeze of the bulb (this is about 18 drops). Use half this amount for a child.

❑ Have the person lay on his side with his head in line with his body. If lying on a bed, you will need to use a pillow, the head should be level with the body, not up higher or lower than the neck and shoulders.

Step 2

❑ Slowly and carefully insert the eye dropper into the ear, and then gently squeeze the bulb 5 or 6 times allowing the liquid from the dropper to go in and out of the ear each time. This should be enough to get the liquid to the bottom of the ear. The goal is to get the liquid to the bottom of the ear. When finished, as the person sits up, soak up the solution that comes out of the ear with a paper towel or tissue and discard. Make up a fresh solution each time you do this procedure.

Notes

> *Normally, especially with children, (because children often heal quicker than adults) this procedure will eliminate most pain immediately, but if not, continue with this procedure hourly until the pain is gone.*

> *The pain may subside, but you should continue with this process 2 to 3 times a day until completely well (free of any infection), which should be from one day to no more than a week.*

Nose

Note: *The formula of the ratio of activated drops to water is different for ears and nose than that of the eyes.*

MMS1 Formula for the Nose (this is the same formula as for the ears)

❑ Activate 1 drop of MMS with 1 drop of 4% HCl, or 50% citric acid. Be sure you have waited the correct amount of time (30 seconds) and that the MMS1 liquid has turned amber in color.

❑ Add 1 ounce/30 ml of distilled or purified water to the 1 activated drop.

❑ This is the basic formula for the nose—1 activated drop to 1 ounce/30 ml of purified water. This will last about one week if kept in a bottle with a tight lid and stored in a cool dark place. So be sure to make up a fresh batch each week if needed.

MMS1 Nose Procedure

The following procedure is effective when a person's nose is stuffed up, and/or when he has a cold. In addition, this same method will usually work when someone has ongoing sinus troubles and a continuously stuffy nose for weeks or even years. This same technique can be used in addition to Protocol 1000 while overcoming the flu.

Step 1

❑ Use the above formula—1 activated drop of MMS to 1 ounce/30 ml of water.

❑ Lay flat on your back on a bed. Do not put your head on a pillow.

Step 2

❑ Put 4 to 8 drops of this solution into one nostril. It will burn a bit as the nose will burn even with plain water, but MMS1 will not do any damage. The idea is to allow some of the MMS1 to drain into your sinuses, and stay there for approximately five minutes. You can expect some of this to run out when you stand up. It helps to have a tissue on hand.

❑ Repeat the above step for the other nostril.

Note: *Do this 3 times a day until you are well which should not be more than four days in most cases. In the event you are not well in four days, continue until you are well.*

Bath and Foot Bath Protocol

Bathing in MMS1 or MMS2 is one more method of getting MMS1 (which produces chlorine dioxide, ClO_2), or MMS2 (which when mixed with water produces hypochlorous acid [HOCl] which is an acid the body uses to destroy pathogens), into the body, albeit by a different route, so it can reach other areas and get deeper into tissues.

Instructions for MMS1 Baths

Full Bath

Note: *For MMS baths do not use water with chlorine or fluoride in it.* *Try to find out if your tap water contains chlorine or fluoride; if it does, use a reverse osmosis water filter or buy purified water in large bottles. Another possible option is that many people say borax can eliminate fluoride and chlorine from bath water. There is much anecdotal evidence on the internet and some chemistry indicates that the boron in borax creates boron fluoride from the fluoride in the water. This is not a poisonous chemical and not dangerous to your health. A similar nonpoisonous chemical is produced from the chlorine as well. Use two rounded tablespoons of borax for a standard size bathtub. Wait at least 15 minutes after stirring the borax into the water, (cold or hot water is OK), then add your MMS.*

Step 1

❑ Activate 20 MMS drops, count to 30 seconds and make sure it has turned amber color.

❑ Add the activated drops to a tub which has 6 to 12 inches (15 to 30 cm) of water. Use hot water, as hot as you can comfortably stand.

❑ Get in the bath and lay down, or try to situate yourself to get as much water on you as possible. If you are not totally submersed, use your hands to gently lap the water up over your body.

❏ Stay in the water for about 20 minutes.

Note: *Begin by using 20 activated MMS drops per bath, the next time use 40 activated drops and then 60.*

Step 2

❏ Take an MMS1 bath 1 to 3 times a day and generally not more than 60 drops per bath.

Step 3

❏ On the second or third day, begin to add DMSO drops to the MMS1 solution after the activation time has completed. (**Be sure that your tub is completely clean and free of any residue from soap**, etc.) At first use 1/2 as many drops of DMSO as activated MMS drops, and then each time you prepare a bath, increase the drops of DMSO until you are using 3 drops of DMSO for every 1 drop of activated MMS (MMS1). It is not necessary to use more than 3 drops of DMSO for each activated drop of MMS. (Keep in mind that when we say 1 drop of MMS1, this is 1 drop of activated MMS. Technically, 1 drop of MMS1 is 2 drops of liquid, [1 drop MMS + 1 drop activator acid = 2 drops of liquid]. However, we refer to this as a 1-drop dose of MMS1. In this case, we do not count the drop of activator. So a 3-drop dose of MMS1 would require 9 drops of DMSO, which is 3 drops of DMSO for every 1 drop of MMS1 [activated MMS].)

❏ Whether you are taking a bath with just MMS1, or you have added DMSO to the water, stay in the water for about 20 minutes.

Notes

➤   Baths can be very important and if you notice feeling better, do not stop taking MMS1 baths (up to three baths a day) until you are sure there is nothing more to be gained.

➤   The instructions above, which suggest taking up to three MMS1 baths a day, and to add DMSO to the bath on the second or third day, is particularly recommended in this amount, in the case of those who are fighting a specific illness and/or life threatening disease. However, the MMS1 bath (or MMS2 bath—see below), can serve many purposes. These baths are great for a general detoxification, especially if one knows they have been "exposed" to some hard hitting toxins, such as due to traveling/airplane flights, or due to spending one or several days in a large polluted city, or being in any overall toxic environment. If you feel the need for some extra detoxification because of what you have been exposed to, then try an MMS bath.

➤   If you happen to live and work in a large polluted city, you might want to consider taking an MMS bath 1 to 3 times a week. Or, you might want to enjoy these baths a few times a week simply for the pleasure of relaxation, and to beautify the skin.

➤   An MMS bath can serve as a beauty treatment and many have reported clearer, smoother and softer skin after adding MMS baths to their weekly schedule. Try the MMS1 or MMS2 bath, see what your body can handle, then add these baths to your routine as the need arises and/or as you feel led.

Foot Bath

A full MMS bath is much more effective and thus more desirable than an MMS foot bath. This is because more of the skin is in direct contact with the MMS solution and various parts of the body have a chance to get the MMS directly through the skin on a targeted area. For example, if you have breast cancer and can immerse yourself (and breasts) under the water, it may be of benefit. Or, if the problem is in the private parts and you are immersed in the MMS water, more can be absorbed directly to the problem area.

For those who may not have a bathtub, or who are unable to get in and out of a tub for one reason or another, or who perhaps do not have enough uncontaminated water for a full bath, I suggest a foot bath. Foot baths are a wonderful way to relax, and with this method a good amount of MMS can still get into the system and do some good. Please note, I suggest the same amount of drops for a foot bath as a full body bath. This is because the skin on the feet, ankles and even the legs tends to be stronger or tougher than the chest, back, arms, stomach and private parts.

Step 1

❑ Use ankle high water in a small plastic basin.

❑ Follow the same directions given above for the full bath with the same amount of MMS1 and DMSO drops.

Variations

➤ If water is scarce, you can prepare the foot bath with little water, not even enough to reach the top of the foot. Put a cloth on top of the foot, and let the water soak into the cloth while some water still remains under the foot. This serves as a type of compress and it will still help more MMS to get into the skin/tissues.

➤ Prepare the foot bath using a deeper recipient for the water, such as a bucket, so the water reaches up to the calf or to the knees. Follow the same formula—add up to 60 activated drops of MMS per bath. This allows a larger skin area to be covered.

Instructions for MMS2 Baths

Caution: Unlike the MMS1 bath, **never ever add DMSO to an MMS2 bath!** (For more details see warning on pages 23-24.)

Step 1

❑ Make up your bath or foot bath water as per the directions in the note in the Full Bath section, page 143.

Step 2

❑ **For a full bath** use 3 level teaspoons (15 ml) of MMS2 (calcium hypochlorite) the first time. If the skin does OK, you can cautiously increase up to 10 level teaspoons (50 ml) of MMS2 per bath. You may want to sprinkle the MMS2 granules into the water without touching them, then once in the water mix it around with your hand. If you do get some of the dry granules on your hands, be careful not to touch your eyes until it is thoroughly rinsed off.

❑ **For a foot bath** use the same measurements as the MMS2 full bath as outlined above.

Note: *Skin types vary widely from person to person. If you notice any irritation or burning of the skin immediately get out of the water and rinse off. The next time use only 1/2 as much MMS2.*

Variation: The same variations listed above for the MMS1 bath can apply for the MMS2 baths, with the exception, again, that you **never, ever add DMSO to an MMS2 bath as the two are not compatible.**

Enema Protocol

Enemas have been used for thousands of years in many cultures to clean the body, alleviate fevers, and heal from illness. It was a commonly used tool of doctors until recent times. It can also be an effective delivery system for MMS1, especially when one has reached the maximum tolerable oral dose.

Using an MMS1 enema is often very important to the recovery of health. The enema delivers chlorine dioxide to the liver and to the bloodstream, as well as neutralizing toxins and killing parasites in the bowel. In addition, adding MMS1 in the enema kills pathogens in the colon and much of the MMS1 is absorbed through the colon walls into the blood plasma. In many cases the enema will give the colon a much needed cleaning.

If you do not know how to give yourself an enema, please study and familiarize yourself with the process before attempting it. There are many instructional sites on the internet for this purpose. Simply put the words "enema how to" into any search engine and you will find all the information you need.

Most enema equipment or kits come with a stiff nozzle which is inserted into the rectum and up into the colon about 6 to 8 inches. As an alternative to using the stiff enema nozzle, I highly suggest using a simple catheter with the enema bag in place of the hard plastic nozzle. The catheter is a flexible tube and thus can help avoid possibly puncturing a hole into the side of the colon, as some have done, using the more rigid tip. Whatever equipment you decide to use, go slow and do not proceed if there is discomfort. (Some enema bags include the catheter tube as well, or they can be purchased separately along with a connector which joins the catheter to the enema bag tube. This equipment is available in most pharmacies, or online for a greater selection.)

Instructions for Enema Protocol

Notes

➤ *Whether you are using enemas on their own for various problems, such as bladder difficulties, or whether you are on other protocols at the same time, 5 drops of activated MMS in 1000 ml (1 liter/quart) of purified water (warm or body temperature) in the enema bag would be a good amount to start with. Increase the drops in each enema until you reach 30 drops. If at any time you feel discomfort or that the solution is too strong, cut the drops in half and work up again slowly from there to what you are comfortable with.*

➤ *Using citric acid as the activator acid can tend to burn if one goes up very high with their drops, especially past 20 drops. For enemas, 4% HCl (hydrochloric acid) is the preferred activator acid to use.*

➤ *Do not use a stainless steel enema bag. Some people consider these the very best, however, stainless steel may react chemically with MMS and therefore is not a good choice.*

Caution: *Never* use DMSO in an enema! Why? The colon contains many toxins the body is flushing out. If you put DMSO in the colon, you can return some of those toxins back into the blood stream.

Step 1

❑ Prepare the water for your enema bag by warming 1000 ml (1 liter/quart) of distilled, reverse osmosis or bottled water to body temperature. (It is important to warm the enema bag water to body temperature, as using cool water could cause severe cramping.)

❑ Select the number of drops you want to use (5 drops the first time). In a clean, dry glass activate your drops and count 30 seconds. (Remember, if using citric acid, you will not want to go past 20 drops per enema. HCl 4% is the preferred activator for enemas.)

❑ Add the activated drops to the warm water you have prepared. Pour some of the warm water into the MMS activating glass and then pour that solution back into the container with the warm water. You now have your enema bag solution. (Be diligent to make sure all utensils used for this preparation are very clean.)

Step 2

❑ Fill your enema bag with the solution. For the first several enemas it is acceptable to use one half of this solution or even less in your enema bag if you are not comfortable using more. You can increase the amount of liquid a little bit each time until you are using the full amount of 1000 ml (1 liter/quart) of solution. Go at your own pace, do not make yourself excessively uncomfortable. Stop before you reach 1000 ml (1 liter/quart) if you feel uncomfortable.

Step 3

❑ Begin the enema. Let the water flow. Try to hold it in for 5 to 10 minutes if you can. If you cannot hold it, that is not a problem. Try holding a smaller amount, it's sometimes easier, then repeat.

Notes

➤   If you start with a 5-drop solution, do that once or twice and then do a 10-drop solution, and so on.

➤   You can go as high as 20 to 30 drops **if you work up to it**, but do not continue if it causes problems.

➤   You can do 2 to 3 enemas a day.

➤   If you see improvement after doing 4 or 5 enemas, keep doing enemas until there is no further indication of improvement. But if there is no improvement after 4 or 5 enemas, do not continue with them. As I said, enemas can be a very important part of health recovery; however, I do not suggest prolonged use of enemas as they can be hard on the body. In this case, if you do not see any signs of progress after 4 or 5 enemas, do not continue. Go on to the next protocol or procedure outlined in the Health Recovery Plan.

Exception: If you are on other protocols and fighting a life-threatening disease, you can increase the drops in the enema accordingly. For example, if you are one of those people who is tolerating a larger amount of MMS1—say you are taking 9 to 12 drops or more an hour in your oral dose—then you may be able to increase the amount of MMS1 you put in your enema bag. But do not go beyond 60 drops in 1000 ml (1 liter/quart) of water per enema. Remember, this is the exception, not the rule.

Good results have been obtained with prostate and bladder problems with enemas, as well as many other problems.

Colonics

A colonic (also called colonic hydrotherapy or colon irrigation) is the infusion of water into the rectum by a colon therapist to cleanse and flush out the colon. Colonics and enemas both aim to cleanse the colon by introducing water by way of the rectum. Although the two methods are similar in approach and in their health benefits, there are some distinct differences between colonics and enemas.

Enemas involve a one-time infusion of water into the colon. Colonics involve multiple infusions of water into the colon. The main objective of enemas is to evacuate the lower colon, while colonics are meant to cleanse a larger part of the colon. The colonic is more thorough and may be more beneficial depending on what the problem and illness is.

Unlike enemas, which can be performed at home with the help of do-it-yourself kits, colonics require specialized equipment and must be administered by a trained colon therapist.

During the colonic warm, filtered water is slowly released into the colon. The water causes the muscles of the colon to contract, called peristalsis. Peristalsis "pushes" feces out through the hose to be disposed in a closed waste system. During this process, the colon therapist may apply light massage to the client's abdominal area to facilitate the process.

You'll want to find an experienced colonics therapist that knows what she/he is doing. The therapist should ask you questions about your health history to be sure there are no contraindications for you to receive the colonics. In addition, the therapist should perform a simple external check of the colon and intestine, as well as a very simple rectal exam to be sure conditions are right for you to receive the colonics.

You'll also want to find a therapist who will use MMS1 in the colonic at your recommendation. They may or may not be experienced with MMS1 (you can direct them on how to use the drops). Be sure to double check that they are using good water and not water from the faucet as it will generally have chlorine and/or fluoride in it. Routinely they will have you put on a gown and lay on a table for the colonic.

I suggest that you use 20 drops of MMS1 (activated MMS) for the first time and 50 drops of MMS1 the second time. If all goes well and you continue with colonics, you can go up to 100 MMS1 drops for subsequent colonic sessions. (This amount of drops is for 20 to 25 liters/quarts of water. If more water is used in the colonic the drops can be adjusted accordingly.)

Remember, there is a lot of water used in a colonic, so this amount of MMS1 is not a problem.

Douche Protocol

This protocol is recommended for vaginal problems, bad infections, as well as cancer and most other diseases and problems (such as fibroids, polyps, and cysts) of the female reproductive organs (ovaries, uterus, and breast). In the case of breast cancer, the cervix absorbs the MMS1 and carries it to the lymphatic system and into the breast. MMS1 in the douche will kill pathogens in the area allowing the body to create health there. Overall, douches are only necessary when something needs to be corrected.

Instructions for MMS1 Douche

The following instructions assume one knows how to do a douche. If not, please sufficiently educate yourself on the process before following this protocol.

Step 1

❑ You will need a 2 cup/500 ml douche bag. You can use a larger douche bag, but it is not necessary to use more than 2 cups/500 ml of water.

❑ Prepare your solution. Start out with 5 drops of MMS1 to the 2 cups/500 ml of purified, distilled or reverse osmosis water. Like the enema, 4% HCl, is the preferred activator acid to use with a douche, although citric acid 50% can be used. It is best to warm the water for the douche to body temperature.

❑ When doing the douche let water flow in until it starts to run out again, then close the flow. (The tube with your douche bag usually comes with a clamp for opening and closing the water flow.)

❑ Squeeze the pelvic/vaginal muscles to hold it in as long as possible, and then release. Repeat this process until the bag is empty.

Step 2

❑ If you have no adverse reactions, then increase the amount of drops of MMS1 for the next douche.

❑ The next time add 10 activated drops to the water you pour into the douche bag, and keep increasing up to 30 drops as long as there is no pain or problem, but do not use more than 30 drops. Increase to this amount slowly.

Adding DMSO to a Douche

❑ Your douche can be more effective with the use of DMSO, which can help the MMS1 penetrate deeper into the tissues. Add 3 drops of DMSO to every 1 drop of MMS1 you are using in your bag.

Caution: When adding DMSO to a douche it is important that you have a douche bag that is not made from rubber or latex (which is a refined form of rubber). There are various kinds of douche containers available, if you want to add DMSO use one that is made of plastic (including the hose), not of rubber, as the rubber may leach into the body along with DMSO.

Notes

➤ *If you experience burning and/or stinging this is usually an indication that fungus is present. In this case, I suggest doing a clay douche. Use 1 level teaspoon of clay (Aztec clay, bentonite, clay, or montmorillonite clay) in 2 cups of water for your douche. Keep the douche container well shook up for these clay douches. Do two or three clay douches a day and always "wash out" the clay (using the douche bag and clean water) after one hour. After three days you can check to see if the fungus is gone by using the same MMS1 solution that initially caused the burning and/or stinging. If you no longer feel stinging and/or burning, this means that the fungus is gone but further non-clay douches may be needed. You can continue with your MMS1 douches as per the instructions in this Douche Protocol.*

➤ *In case of cancer or bad infections you can douche 4 to 5 times a day (work up to this). Be sure that the douching does not cause irritation.*

> *Normally, douche 1 to 4 times a day, depending on the severity of the problem. One time a day may be enough. It is up to you to determine how many times each day. Remember the rule, as long as you are improving do not stop, but don't continue if there is no benefit.*

> *Do your last douche of the day before bedtime for absorption and detoxing as you sleep. Remember, if after about a week you do not see any improvement, do not continue, but do continue as long as there is improvement.*

> *Anytime you are doing the Douche Protocol, it is always a good idea to be taking the oral protocol, either Protocol 1000, or Protocol 2000, depending on the situation.*

MMS Bag Protocol

This process in an additional way to get MMS1 (chlorine dioxide) into and on the body, helping to overcome pathogens, poisons and heavy metals. This gassing process is more intense than using a spray bottle.

Caution: Avoid breathing in any of the fumes. Controlled skin contact of MMS1 is ok, but your lungs can not tolerate much chlorine dioxide gas. Open a window in the room while you are doing this. If you happen to breathe in a few breaths of MMS1 fumes, you may not have much of a reaction at first, but should you breathe it in, it is possible that some time later (four hours or so), you may experience difficulty in breathing for awhile. It is best to avoid directly breathing it in to begin with.

Instructions for MMS1 Bag Protocol

This procedure can be done 2 times a day, over a period of a few days if needed. One will need to start out with a certain number of activated drops and build up the amount over three days. Be sure to carefully read and have a good understanding of each point below before attempting this protocol.

Step 1

❑ Take two large garbage bags (the big black ones work best) and make one bag out of them. Lay them on a table, or on the floor, join them together at the opening of each bag. At this junction tape them all the way around with 2" (5cm) wide shipping/packaging tape so that the mouth of each bag is taped to the other, making one long bag. (You might start by using small pieces of tape to hold them together, and then tape them all the way around with wide tape, taping first one side and then the other.)

❑ Cut one end of the bag open, and then check to see that it is not stuck together in the center where you taped the two bags together.

Step 2

❑ Undress completely, or use as little clothing as possible.

❑ Open the bag and step into it. At this point it helps to have a chair handy, so you can sit down. With your feet in the bag, pull it up to about waist high, then sit down on the chair and prepare your drops.

❑ On the first day, put 20 drops of MMS and 20 drops of 50% citric acid or 4% HCl in a cup, and immediately (don't wait to count 30 seconds) set the cup inside the bag so that it rests on the floor near your feet, being careful not to let it spill. If it does spill be careful not to get it on your feet, but go ahead and use it as it will create chlorine dioxide fumes just as well.

❑ Carefully stand up and pull the bag up around your shoulders and neck, wrapping and folding the plastic so that no fumes escape.

Caution: Do not put your head inside the bag or breathe any of the fumes.

Step 3

❑ The first day, stay in the bag five minutes, no longer. If you feel any burning sensation on your skin, get out of the bag immediately, even if five minutes has not passed. (In this case, rinse off and/or shower.)

❑ Repeat this entire procedure 1 more time the first day, (in other words, 2 times a day).

Step 4

❑ As long as there is no irritation to skin, do this procedure for two more days. On the second day use 30 activated drops, and on the third day use 40 activated drops. As long as there is no irritation to the skin, you can extend the time in the bag up to 10 minutes, but no longer. If you feel any burning sensation on your skin, get out of the bag immediately and shower off. With or without a burning sensation, **do not surpass 10 minutes in the bag.** There is no need to shower after this process unless there is a burning sensation.

Step 5

❑ If things are going well, you can keep it up for a few more days until you can determine if it is helping or not. If you notice improvement, keep it up as long as it is helping.

Notes

➤   *Use this protocol for skin problems, or to simply get more MMS into your body. If it is helping, remember, keep it up!*

➤   *You cannot use CDS or CDH for this protocol.*

Lung Protocol (The Cup)

It is important to note that **this protocol must be followed explicitly.** Please make sure you read this protocol all the way through a couple of times, and that you have a clear understanding of each step, before you even attempt to do it. Chlorine dioxide gas by itself, as it is used in this procedure, is the strongest way we ingest it. Therefore I cannot stress enough the need to **closely heed the instructions** or it can otherwise be dangerous. Likewise, if you will **carefully follow the instructions** it can also breathe new life into your lungs.

If you follow these instructions to the letter there is no danger, but people often get too enthusiastic and do too much and then they can suffer. I hesitate to tell the world about this protocol, not because of what I tell you here, but because enthusiastic people sometimes overdo it because they want to get well quickly. Some may take what I say here and carry it too far. So **go slow and do not overdo it.** In this case more is definitely not better.

Lung Problems

I can give you many names of diseases for lungs: asthma, COPD, cystic fibrosis, bacterial pneumonia, emphysema, pulmonary embolism, and mild to serious respiratory diseases of all kinds, such as the common cold, croup, tuberculosis and lung cancer. Most diseases of the lungs cause symptoms you can feel, and many of them will make you cough. Coughing generally is not caused by a tickling in the throat but mainly because the body is trying to cough up mucus that tends to block the breathing tubes. Mucus can also hide various diseases. Getting rid of mucus in the lungs is key to curing the lungs. This protocol, which I like to call "the cup" is for that purpose. In addition to getting rid of mucus, the chlorine dioxide gas released from the MMS1 (activated MMS) can also kill disease pathogens in the lungs which are not hiding in mucus.

How to Help Your Lungs with MMS1 Gas (using the cup)

Step 1

❑ Use a clean, dry cup or glass that holds 8 ounces of liquid. (A glass that is about 3 inches/7.6cm in diameter at the top is ideal.) **Absolutely do not use a metal cup** as it will react negatively with the mixture.

❑ Activate 2 drops of MMS with 2 drops of 50% citric acid or 4% HCl. Immediately hold your hand across the mouth of the cup, completely covering it, and count 10 seconds. (While counting, swirl the drops in the cup slightly to mix them well.)

Step 2

❑ After 10 seconds, bring the cup up to your nose slowly and then remove your hand. Putting your nose right over the brim of the cup, **breathe in slowly** until you feel a "bite" (a stinging or smarting sensation) at the end of your nose. **Once you feel a bite, stop immediately.** Do this only one time, breathing through the nose.

Step 3

❏ Then put your hand over the mouth of the cup again for another 10 seconds.

❏ After the second 10-second count, bring the cup up to your mouth, remove your hand from the cup and **breathe in slowly** through your mouth from the mouth of the cup until you begin to feel a "bite" in your lungs, then stop.

That's it for this session.

Remember

- When breathing through the nose and through the mouth—breathe slowly.

- You want to be especially careful to only breathe deep enough to *begin* to feel a bite (a stinging or smarting sensation). The key is to get to that point, but no more.

- The onset of the bite is the signal to stop.

Step 4

❏ After eight to ten hours or so, repeat Steps 1 through 3 as outlined above. Do this procedure only **2 times a day**, once in the morning and once in the evening.

What to Look For

Probably the most important thing to look for and to keep in mind while doing this process is that MMS is supposed to make you feel better, not worse. If you are feeling worse when using this Lung Protocol, something is wrong, and you should back off. Lower the amount of drops in the cup to 1 drop of MMS1, breathe in a little less or stop altogether for a time. Just go slowly until you are feeling better.

Important Points for The Cup Procedure

1. When following the cup procedure: If you have a serious lung condition, you should also be doing the MMS protocols. Normally you would begin with the Starting Procedure and work on up to Protocol 1000, Protocol 1000 Plus, and proceed to Protocol 2000 if needed (according to the Health Recovery Plan as outlined in this book). Remember, **build up your dosing slowly.**

2. Follow all the instructions: The **timing** of this procedure and the size of the cup or glass you use **is extremely important.** The cup/glass should be at least 8 ounces (approximately 250 ml), a little over this capacity is OK, but get it as close to 8 ounces as possible. This is the preferred size to be able to create enough gas inside the cup. The **10-second count is also very important,** as if you wait much longer the amount of gas to be inhaled will be stronger, and may be too much to take at once. As I mentioned above, please **follow these directions explicitly**.

3. Coughing: You can have a coughing fit anywhere from immediately after breathing the cup up to several hours or even a day after doing this procedure. This is normal, as the chlorine dioxide gas is working on breaking up mucus and it needs to be expelled. It will loosen some of the mucus that forms in your lungs that can hold pathogens. This mucus will then either run down into your stomach and slowly work its way out of your system, or your body will cough the mucus up and you will be able to spit it out. You may cough long and hard, possibly up to an hour or so, to just get a little tiny bit of mucus up—this is part of the process. You may find that huge amounts of mucus will come out through your nose, so have plenty of tissue on hand.

In the case of a coughing spell that won't stop, if it continues more than an hour, you may need to loosen some more of the mucus that is holding on too tight (stuck to the sides of the breathing tubes). In this particular case, you might feel a little worse due to the coughing. The next step in this case is to begin taking Aztec clay, bentonite clay, or montmorillonite clay. Take one level teaspoon of the clay in 1/2 cup of water or appropriate juice every hour for three or four hours until the coughing stops.

With this particular procedure, when you are awake, you will usually cough up mucus that has been freed from your lungs or breathing tubes, but when you sleep the mucus often drains down into your stomach, and that is not bad. Your body will take care of it with your own stomach acid and process it through your system, and it will not hurt you.

Notes

➤ *If the coughing spells mentioned above (which can occur after breathing the cup) last longer than a one-hour period, this is an indication you need to reduce the drops in the cup to 1 drop rather than 2 drops.*

➤ *If coughing has reached the point of nothing coming up, go to the Cough Protocol (page 131) and follow the directions there.*

4. Catching a cold: It is possible to catch a cold while doing this protocol. This is because mucus drains from the lungs, and on rare occasions it can release cold germs that were protected by mucus. If you catch a cold, simply continue with the process and it should go away in a day or two providing you are also taking MMS1 or MMS2 orally as per Protocol 1000 or 2000 according to your need.

5. Go slowly: The lung process is something you can easily overdo. But remember, one of my golden rules: As long as you are getting better, don't change what you are doing. If your condition seems to get worse, stop or do smaller amounts of MMS. Keep it up until your lungs are healthy. Remember, go easy. And use clay (as mentioned above in point 3 on coughing) when needed.

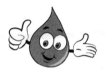

Bronchitis: I suffered with a severe case of bronchitis every year in the winter for 5 years in a row. I found MMS and started taking it at the first sign of symptoms. I haven't had bronchitis in over 3 years now. I take it once a week during cold season just as prevention and every time anyone in our household shows any symptoms of cold, flu, etc., we grab the MMS and start dosing. It works every time. —M. R., United States

Breathe Easy: I've been a smoker for many years. When I mix up a batch of MMS and start taking the 3 drop dose in 4 ounces of water, my breathing is so much easier. If you have any breathing problems or lung congestion, start taking 3 drops of MMS every hour. —B. S., United States

Eczema: I found that MMS has totally cleared up the facial eczema I have suffered with very badly for two years. I tried everything, nothing worked but within days MMS knocked it on the head. Amazing. —Peter, New Zealand

Chapter 10

Indian Herb – The Ultimate Health Recovery Effort

If, after doing all of the protocols outlined in the Health Recovery Plan you have not recovered your health, then using Indian Herb is the next course of action. However, before you go on to this final procedure please carefully consider, once again, the list of possible reasons why you may not be having complete success with MMS thus far. (See Chapter 8, Reality Check.)

This procedure might be a very important part of recovering one's health. There are some cases where it seems that MMS is not helping a tumor to shrink. This might be temporary, but maybe not. After using Protocols 1000, 1000 Plus, 2000, 3000, Mold/Fungus, and all the various Supporting Protocols described in this book as they apply, if sufficient progress is not seen, only then is it time to consider taking Indian Herb.

Indian Herb has helped thousands of people over the past 80 years. This salve does not work the same way MMS does, so expect different side effects. This herbal blend may cause pain, swelling, itching and sometimes fever, thus we prefer MMS. However, there are people alive today who would not otherwise be here had they not used Indian Herb. Many people have used pain relievers in order to withstand the pain of the herb, but many did not.

Instructions for Indian Herb

Step 1

❑ Do not stop taking MMS. Continue with all the various things you have added on to your protocol: MMS1, MMS2, DMSO, enemas, baths, etc. In other words continue with everything you have already been using.

Step 2

❑ Include Indian Herb as part of what you are already doing. You can order it from Kathleen (McDaniel Life-Line Water) at:

http://www.lifelinewater.com

Step 3

❑ Follow the instructions sent with Indian Herb.

The instructions suggest that you dilute it with 4 parts Vaseline to 1 part Indian Herb. In some tough heavy cases if the Indian Herb is not doing the job when mixed with Vaseline, you may have to use the herb full strength. Only use it full strength after you have tried the suggested 4-to-1 mixture. Please note, the stronger the mixture, the more pain you will experience.

In other words, you could use as much as double the amount that is given in the instructions, and as strong as full strength Indian Herb. But do not use full strength right off, as the lesser amount (4-to-1) will probably do the job and also give less pain. (You could also try a stronger 2-to-1 mixture, if the 4-to-1 is not getting results to see if it helps before going to full-strength.)

Step 4

❑ For cancer inside the body one should take Indian Herb orally. We generally use a #1 size vegetable or gel capsule filled 1/2 full, but to start, only fill to 1/4 full and take it twice a day. Follow the instructions that come with Indian Herb but please observe the comments above. When taking Indian herb orally, space it out from your MMS doses by two hours.

Black Salve

Black Salve sold by Adrian Jones, in Australia, is similar to the Indian Herb mentioned above–almost the same in-structions apply. The main ingredient in this salve is the same as in Indian Herb, and that is zinc chloride. The other ingredients are very strong herbs and only two of the four herbs are different from the Indian Herb formula. If you obtain Black Salve from Adrian, be sure to follow his instructions to the letter. If for some reason you did not have Adrian's instruction sheets it would be accept-able to follow the Indian Herb instructions and vice versa.

There are other somewhat similar healing salve formulas available. The terms "Black Salve" and "Indian Herb" often relate to cancer salves in general. There are many different recipes for different purposes. When I say Indian Herb and Black Salve, I am referring to Indian Herb from Kathleen, and Black Salve from Adrian Jones, as these are the two formulas that I am familiar with. I have used Indian Herb extensively to overcome cancers. Indian Herb has been sold by Kathleen in Texas, and her father before her, for over 70 years. She has received hundreds of letters telling of success against cancers and other tumors. Black Salve by Adrian Jones has had much similar success.

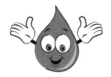

Gall Bladder: My son (24) was admitted to hospital with a blocked bile duct and gall stones. He was in a lot of pain and could not eat as he brought it all back up. The doctors wanted to take his gall bladder out but he refused because it is there for a purpose. He was in hospital for 10 days because the doctors did not appear to want to take the blockage out without the gall bladder. He was also very jaundiced. I stayed with him the whole time because I was [carefully] giving him MMS every hour...They took blood tests every day and on the ninth day they said he had pancreatitis (life threatening) and they would be operating in the morning. That afternoon he passed the blockage and started to feel a lot better. In the morning when they took a blood test everything was dropping to normal. They still went in to remove the blockage but it had gone. Instead they put a stent in to help drain all the rubbish that was still left behind. When he went back in three months the gall stones had disappeared too. He has not had any more problems with his gall bladder. —Ruth B., Australia

❧❧

Diabetes: Thank you kindly, it is a wonderful product, the grandfather is now off his diabetes pills (so many of them) and is so much happier and so full of life again. It is a miracle product. —Nikki

❧❧

Brain Fog: I've been taking MMS, though not steadily, for about 5 months and my head has cleared up...I feel much clearer now, and less brain fog! —N

Chapter 11

Additional Protocols

Protocol 6 and 6

Protocol 6 and 6 is something that can be used on its own—separate from all the other protocols. This protocol consists of taking a 6-drop dose of MMS1 and waiting one hour and then taking another 6-drop dose of MMS1. The purpose of this protocol is to handle many acute things that seem to pop up from time to time such as colds or flu coming on, headaches, fevers, a touch of food poisoning, or any kind of sickness that seems to be just starting, or immediately after being exposed to a bad disease, or germs. It also has been proven successful with chronic pains, even those that have persisted for many months or years. It should be used immediately after any kind of an accident, the sooner the better, even at the scene of the accident. Protocol 6 and 6 has proven successful in a wide range of situations, therefore we suggest you keep some MMS and acid activator handy at all times, so you can mix up an MMS1 dose whenever needed.

Instructions for Protocol 6 and 6

Step 1

❑ Prepare a 6-drop dose as per the instructions in Activating MMS and Mixing a Basic Dose of MMS1, on page 32. (Be sure the drops turn amber color.)

❑ Add 1/2 cup (4 ounces/120 ml) of water or other approved liquid that is compatible with MMS1 as per the instructions on pages 41-45.

❑ Drink down the 6-drop dose.

Step 2

❑ In one hour prepare another 6-drop dose and drink it down.

Step 3

❑ The following hour, after taking your second 6-drop dose, if you are feeling OK, then that's it.

Step 4

❑ If you are not feeling OK by the end of the second hour, it is time to get started on the Key Protocols of the Health Recovery plan—begin with the Starting Procedure (see page 79). From the time you took your last 6-drop dose (of Protocol 6 and 6), start with 1/4-drop doses each hour for the rest of the day.

Step 5

❑ The next day (day two), go right into the second day of the Starting Procedure, which is taking 1/2-drop doses every hour for eight hours.

❑ Continue on to complete days three and four of the Starting Procedure.

Step 6

❑ When finished with the Starting Procedure, proceed from there on to Protocol 1000 and continue with the HRP as needed (see Chapter 5).

Note: *Protocol 6 and 6 often handles a variety of on-coming illnesses quickly by destroying pathogens before they are able to get a strong hold in the body. However, we have found that when these first two 6-drop doses do not nip the problem in the bud, then it is best to go to hourly doses according to the HRP (see Chapter 5). Con-tinuing to take 6-drop doses every hour, will likely cause a Herxheimer reaction, and this will slow healing in the long-run. So, if after two 6-drop doses you are not well, begin the Starting Procedure and continue with the HRP as needed.*

Protocol 4000

This protocol entails using MMS2 (calcium hypochlorite) on its own, that is, without using MMS1 at the same time. Protocol 4000 is not used in the line-up of the HRP (Health Recovery Plan) as the next step after Protocol 3000, which one might think its name implies. It was originally meant to be used mostly in emergencies when sodium chlorite (MMS) was not available.

Protocol 4000 is basically taking 5 capsules of MMS2 a day.

Instructions for Protocol 4000

Step 1

❑ Make up some MMS2 capsules and follow the procedures on how to increase your doses as per the instructions in Protocol 2000, Steps 3 and 4 (see page

93). The first day take a total of 5 capsules of MMS2. Fill the first 2 capsules as suggested in Step 3 and then continue increasing the amount slowly according to the instructions in Step 4. (See also MMS2—Details, page 274.)

Step 2

❑ Once you have reached the maximum size dose, continue taking 5 capsules of MMS2 a day. Space out each dose by two hours.

Step 3

❑ Do this for 21 days or until well. Be sure to follow the Three Golden Rules of MMS.

Notes

➤   *Remember, in case of nausea or diarrhea reduce the amount of calcium hypochlorite in each capsule by 50%. When these symptoms subside, slowly increase the amount to the suggested amounts given on page 94.*

➤   ***Never take an MMS2 capsule and a dose containing DMSO at the same time!*** *For a full explanation see pages 23-24.*

➤   ***Maintenance for MMS2 capsules****: Take one capsule of the maximum dose given for MMS2 on page 94 one time (either in the morning or in the evening), every day for maintenance. If you have not taken MMS2 prior to beginning a maintenance dose with it, work up gradually to this suggested dosage.*

Vaccine Procedure

To the best of my knowledge, based on 22 years of working with MMS, I believe that MMS can help avoid vaccine injuries when the process described below is followed. From all the thousands of people who have used MMS there is ample evidence that MMS removes poisons, toxins and kills pathogens that cause disease. According to information sheets included with vaccines, most vaccines contain these very things. Therefore it stands to reason MMS would be effective in neutralizing any possible negative side effects of vaccines, used within minutes, hours, or even several days after the vaccination. (However, doing it as soon as possible after the vaccination is best.)

Many people are concerned about possible vaccine injuries, and a growing number of parents do not want their children to be subjected to them. Therefore I want to present the following procedure. Included is the MMS1/DMSO Patch Protocol, which we have found to be very effective in neutralizing skin poisons and toxins.

Those of you in the US, and other countries where possible, may want to investigate how to claim *religious exemption* from vaccines. However, if you are in a position where you have no choice but to take a vaccination, you may want to try this protocol.

Note: *I suggest this procedure be followed using MMS1 drops mixed fresh hourly, not other forms of MMS (CDS or CDH).*

Instructions for Vaccine Procedure—Dosing for Adults

Two Weeks Before a Vaccination

❑ Do the Starting Procedure, followed by Protocol 1000 (see pages 79-87).

Day of the Vaccine

❑ Take 6 drops of MMS1 (activated MMS) every two hours, (for a total of 4 times) during an eight-hour period. Begin this dosing one to two hours before you get the vaccine.

❑ **Immediately after the vaccination** is injected (preferably when you get back to your car, or the moment you get home—though the sooner the better), do the MMS1/DMSO Patch Protocol (see page 135). The MMS1/DMSO Patch will help neutralize the toxins in the vaccine.

❑ Apply this patch 1 more time on vaccination day, three hours after the first application. If you feel the need to apply a third patch in another three hours you may do so. But three patches in total should be sufficient.

Note: *Please be diligent to closely follow the instructions for making an MMS1/DMSO patch on page 135. Add more water to the patch, or discontinue use if there is any burning or irritation. Keep a close watch.*

Day After the Vaccination

❑ Continue Protocol 1000 for one week to make sure all toxins are eliminated from the body.

Notes

➤ *If at any time while taking these doses you begin to feel nausea or diarrhea, lower your intake of MMS1. Cut the amount you are taking in half, then work back up from there when the ill feelings subside.*

➤ *There may be times when you have no warning before getting a vaccine. Sometimes when traveling, vaccinations can be required to enter various countries. If you do not have warning before getting a vaccination, simply start with "Day of the Vaccine" points listed above. In this case, depending upon how your body is reacting, you may want to continue Protocol 1000 for three weeks after the vaccine, instead of one week.*

➤ This same procedure applies to oral vaccinations, with the exception that there would be no need for the MMS1/DMSO Patch Protocol.

Instructions for Vaccine Procedure—Dosing for Children

The Vaccine Procedure for children follows a similar routine as for adults. That is, two weeks before a vaccine begin the protocol. Then there are specific dosing suggestions for the day of the vaccine and further instructions for the day after the vaccine, etc. The amount of MMS1 drops given to children, *must* be adjusted according to the weight of the child.

Adults follow the standard Starting Procedure and Protocol 1000 for much of this procedure for vaccines. In the case of children, I also suggest doing the standard Starting Procedure and Protocol 1000 for children (calculated according to the child's weight) which is listed on pages 256-258. This is as long as there is one or two weeks advance notice before receiving a vaccine. If there is less than one week advance warning, dose the child according to the Vaccine Dosage Chart for Children (below) as many days in advance of the vaccine as possible. Or, if there is no warning you can start with the Day of the Vaccine Chart on the day of the vaccine.

Two Weeks Before a Vaccination

❑ Begin with the Starting Procedure followed by Protocol 1000 for children (pages 256-258), and stick with this until the day of the vaccine.

❑ If you are unable to start one or two weeks in advance, nevertheless begin dosing according to the Vaccine Dosage Chart for Children whenever you can, be it a week in advance, three days in advance, or whatever the case may be.

Vaccine Dosage Chart for Children	
Weight	**MMS1 Dosage**
Babies weighing less than 7 lbs (3.2 kg)	Start them on 1/4 drop per hour the first day, and then 1/2 drop an hour thereafter.
7-24 lbs (3.2-10 kg)	Start them on 1/2 drop per hour for the first day, and 3/4 drop per hour thereafter.
Above 25 lbs (11 kg), the basic rule of thumb is to give 1 drop of MMS1 (activated MMS) for every additional 25 lbs for a child.	
25-49 lbs (11-22 kg)	1 drop per hour
50-74 lbs (22-33 kg)	2 drops per hour
75 lbs (34 kg) and over	3 drops per hour

Day of the Vaccine

❑ Give the child the appropriate amount of MMS1 drops (activated MMS) according to the Day of the Vaccine Chart for Children (see below). Do this every two hours, (for a total of 4 times) during an eight-hour period. Begin this dosing one to two hours before the vaccine is administered.

❑ **Immediately after the vaccination** is injected (preferably when you get back to your car, or the moment you get home—though the sooner the better), do the MMS1/DMSO Patch Protocol (see following page). Or, in the case of a baby or children with very sensitive skin, follow instructions for adjusting the Patch Protocol for babies and people with sensitive skin (see following page). The MMS1/DMSO Patch will help neutralize the toxins in the vaccine.

❑ Apply this patch 1 more time on vaccination day, three hours after the first application. If you feel the need to apply a third patch in another three hours you may do so. But three patches in total should be sufficient.

Note: *Please be diligent to closely follow the instructions for making an MMS1/DMSO patch on page 135. Add more water to the patch, or discontinue use if there is any burning or irritation. Keep a close watch.*

| Day of Vaccine MMS1 Dosages for Children ||
Weight	MMS1 Dosage
Babies under 7 lbs (3.2 kg)	3/4 drop every 2 hours
7-24 lbs (3.2-10 kg)	1 drop every 2 hours
25-49 lbs (11-22 kg)	2 drops every 2 hours
50-74 lbs (22-33 kg)	4 drops every 2 hours.
75 lbs (34 kg) and over	6 drops every 2 hours.

Adjusting the MMS1/DMSO Patch Protocol for Babies and People with Sensitive Skin

Please read and have a good understanding of the instructions for the standard MMS1/DMSO Patch Protocol (page 135). This protocol is basically the same procedure, but the amounts of MMS1 drops/water and the timing for applying the patch is adjusted to accommodate sensitive skin.

❑ Start with 5 drops of MMS1 (activated MMS). Add 5 drops of DMSO and 10 additional drops of water to dilute the solution.

❑ For the very first application do not apply the patch for more than five minutes.

❑ When the patch is removed take note if there is irritation. If there is no irritation after five minutes with the first patch, in two hours apply another patch, this time leave it on for 15 minutes. If there is no skin irritation or burning on the next 15 minute application it is OK to continue with one more application (in the case of a vaccine) if you feel the need.

❑ If at any time there is skin irritation or burning, then double the additional amount of water beyond what was used on the last application.

Day After the Vaccination

❑ Continue dosing the child according to the Vaccine Dosage Chart for Children (page 176) for 1 week to make sure all toxins are eliminated from the body.

Notes

➤ *For instructions on how to measure a fraction of a drop, see the Starting Procedure, page 79.*

➤ **Never exceed the maximum amount of MMS1 per hour for each weight category.**

➤ *Remember, if at any time while taking these doses your child begins to experience nausea or diarrhea, lower the intake of MMS1. Cut the amount in half, then work back up from there when the ill feelings subside.*

Lung Tumor: The good news is that my sister's lung tumor was completely gone after only being on MMS for 40 days! She only took a one drop dose for 8 hours a day. By day 10, she started coughing up the tumor. I'm so very grateful for this amazing information and product! Thanks to all of you for your contribution to helping others regain their health! Blessings to you all! —R.D.

౿∾ଙ

Cataracts: I had cataracts and after taking the MMS for a month, 8 times a day (3 drops each time, in approximately 4 oz of water), plus dropping some of the water into my eyes, it cleared up! —Nancy

౿∾ଙ

Nephritus Recovery: Had nephritus and both my feet swelled up for over two years. Did Protocol 1000 and within 10 days the swelling receded and now my both my feet are back to normal. Thank you Jim. —Andy Z., United States

Malaria Protocol

Malaria is one of the simplest diseases to handle with MMS, as it only requires 1 or 2 doses of MMS1 drops. However, unlike using MMS1 for other ailments, for malaria you give 1 initial very strong dose of activated drops (MMS1), followed by 1 more strong dose an hour or two later. Under other circumstances, you would not normally give such a strong dose, and if you did, the person would likely be nauseous or possibly vomit unless they worked up to this amount slowly. But, with malaria this very rarely happens, and the large dose seems to knock the malaria parasite out in about four hours, normally without nausea or additional sicknesses.

In my past books, I have suggested using a 15-drop dose of MMS1 to handle malaria. But because the malaria parasite seems to vary widely in its ability to withstand oxidation caused by MMS1 (chlorine dioxide) while in the body, I have found the need to adjust this dosing. There still remains only four strains of malaria that affect humans. However, those four strains vary widely in their strength or weakness from region to region and therefore in their resistance to MMS1 oxidation power.

Normally a single dose of 18 activated drops of MMS will kill most malaria strains in an adult, but unfortunately not always. For some malaria areas in the world it takes up to 30 drops in a single dose to knock out malaria, while in other areas it takes as little as 6 drops to totally kill malaria in an adult. As I said above, normally an 18-drop dose will handle most malaria, and this is what I suggest for the basic malaria dose. You wouldn't want to start someone out on a 30-drop dose of MMS1 if it is not needed, as that could make people extremely nauseous.

So, especially when someone is in a malaria area and attempting to help many cases of malaria he/she must determine the minimum dose needed to kill malaria, in their specific region. I will outline how to go about this further along in this section.

The female Anopheles mosquito is the carrier of the malaria parasite. When someone is bitten by a mosquito carrying malaria, the malaria parasites travel to the liver where they multiply and finally make their way into the blood after seven days or longer. When in the blood they begin to take over and destroy red blood cells. This is the point where the victim becomes sick and feels all the symptoms of malaria. One will not feel any symptoms until the malaria travels out of the liver and into the blood. MMS1 can kill the malaria parasites before they leave the liver, or it can kill the parasites in the blood.

When MMS1 is taken orally it seems to have the best effect against malaria. Normally, 98% of all malaria is handled with 2 oral doses of MMS1 and you don't have to go any further in helping the malaria victim. However, I have added extra instructions below for the situation where larger doses are required, and also for the areas that do not require the large doses of 18 drops.

Quick test strips (rapid diagnostic tests for malaria RDTs) which are used to determine if a person has malaria are considered effective. However, the quick test strips cannot be used to tell if a person is malaria free after taking MMS1 or any of the other various treatments for malaria. This is because malaria antigens will be present in the blood for weeks. The antigens are what give a positive reading that may be false. Accurate testing to determine if a person is malaria free involves looking at the blood under a microscope. (See page 185.)

An Ounce of Prevention...

For all those living in, or traveling to, a known malaria region, I highly suggest a daily maintenance dose of MMS1 is in order. Prevention is better than illness. (See page 200 for details on the maintenance dose for both adults and children.)

Instructions for Malaria Protocol

Adults

Step 1

❑ A person should take one 18-drop dose of MMS1 (activated MMS) in 3/4 cup (6 oz or 180 ml) of purified water if possible.

Step 2

❑ Within one to two hours after the first dose, repeat Step 1 above—that is, take another 18-drop dose of MMS1.

Note: *Two 18-drop doses will overcome 90% of all malaria cases. Actually, usually the first 18-drop dose kills the malaria, but I suggest giving a second 18-drop dose just to make sure the malaria is totally gone.* **This is the basic dosing procedure for malaria.**

Additional Actions Which may be Needed for the Basic Malaria Dose

➤ When following the basic dosage for malaria, (given above) if the first 18-drop dose seems to make the malaria victim sicker, this indicates less MMS1 is needed. The person should drink water until the sickness brought on by the MMS1 dose passes, and he should be alright. If his malaria symptoms have not subsided and he is not feeling better, then I suggest he take a second dose of MMS1, but with 25% less drops—that would be a 13-drop dose. Even if his symptoms of malaria are gone after his first 18-drop dose, and even though that dose may have made him a little sicker initially, it would be wise to give him one more 13-drop dose, to be sure all the malaria is eradicated.

➤ If the first 2 doses (either two 18-drop doses or, one 18-drop dose and one 13-drop dose) do not overcome the malaria within a total of four hours, in other words in four hours if the person is not feeling much better, then give a third dose at the end of four hours. This third dose should be 18 drops of MMS1 if the malaria victim experienced no additional sickness with the first two 18-drop doses. Or, if the person already had to go down to a 13-drop dose, as explained in the paragraph above, then give another 13-drop dose for the 3rd dose. After this 3rd dose, wait two hours. If the malaria symptoms are gone then you can assume everything is OK and the individual can go home. (In the event they start feeling bad again the next day, they should return and take more MMS1. There could be a variety of reasons why the person could start feeling bad again. See further explanation below.)

➤ If the malaria symptoms continue after taking 3 doses of MMS1, the victim should continue taking MMS1 every hour, but reduce the dose to 6 drops of MMS1 every hour. If the victim becomes sicker while taking the 6 drops an hour, immediately stop the MMS1; you should not give the person more MMS1 until his added sickness caused by the MMS1 is gone.

➤ In a case where a person had to back off of the 6-drop doses, wait until the added sickness is gone and then he should begin on Protocol 1000 which he should continue by following the instructions in this book, increasing or going to the next protocol as is suggested in the Health Recovery Plan (HRP). He can stop taking MMS1 when the malaria is gone, unless an additional sickness or disease is present which would also indicate continuing to do Protocol 1000 and following the Three Golden Rules of MMS.

Notes

➤ As I mentioned above, the standard MMS1 dosage of two 18-drop doses will most often eradicate malaria. If you find the need to keep giving MMS1 doses, as I have explained above, this may be necessary for a variety of reasons. There can be many factors involved in the equation which would necessitate continuing with MMS1. For example, one major reason could be that the malaria victim also has another disease—or even multiple illnesses—in addition to malaria, and this would require more MMS1, and possibly MMS2.

➤ In addition, keep in mind all the reasons why MMS might not be having an effect as outlined in Chapter 8 of this book. Thankfully, malaria is knocked out very quickly with MMS1, nevertheless the person should not be eating or drinking things that are not compatible with MMS1 while taking their doses and so on. Remember, if MMS1 seems to not be working—there could be many reasons why. So in a case where MMS1 seems to not be working the best course of action would be for the person to start on Protocol 1000 at 1 activated drop per hour and follow through as given in the protocol instructions according to the Health Recovery Plan.

➤ There have been cases where someone still had malaria the next day and it was discovered that they didn't like the taste and spit the dose out without anyone knowing. If the *person doesn't take the whole dose, it may very well not work. This can be a problem with small children who have issues with taste.*

Helping the Masses Recover from Malaria

The following instructions are taking into account that one is in a malaria area of the world with the intention of helping many people recover from malaria. As mentioned above, I have found there are times you must give either a good bit more or less of the standard malaria dose in order to help people recover their health. Again, this is because the different types of malaria seem to be stronger or weaker in different areas due to a number of reasons, which I will not go into here. But the bottom line is, you will want to determine what the standard dose of MMS1 should be for the particular type of malaria that is prevalent in the area you are in.

In a situation where you only have one or two malaria cases to handle, it may not matter if you have to take the time to give your malaria victims several doses—they will get well, though it might take a little bit longer. But in a situation where you may have hundreds or even thousands of people to help, you will want to kill the malaria with the first dose, followed by the second within two hours, as many will not be able to return for more doses for a variety of reasons. Therefore it is best to take care of it as quickly as possible. This is the main and very important reason why I recommend you determine what dosage to start with so as to knock out malaria quickly in any given region.

Microscope

Many people who set out to help eliminate malaria think they must have a microscope to determine if malaria is present, and when it is eliminated. It would be nice if one were to have a microscope and a technician to determine if the malaria is completely gone, but unfortunately in Africa and many places of the world this is not always possible because of finances and other reasons. If you have a microscope and can determine the presence or absence of malaria in the blood that is helpful, but it is a long way from being an absolute necessity.

Believe me, in malaria areas of the world, people know if they have malaria or not. They live with it year after year; unfortunately, it is a part of their lives. They know when they are sick with it, and they know when they feel well. So, determine how the person is feeling, because when using MMS if one is feeling much better, it is normally a clear indication that they have overcome malaria. This may not be true with other malaria drugs, but after taking MMS1 and the malaria victim says he is feeling good, you can be pretty sure he is malaria free. When using the microscope you will have to wait 24 hours to prove that all the malaria is gone, while only about four hours is necessary by simply asking the person how he is feeling. It has been my experience after helping thousands of malaria victims, that when the person is feeling good after taking the second dose of MMS, you can be pretty sure that he is malaria free.

Many people that feel good go home after four hours and never come back. However, after taking MMS1, a micro-scope test after only four hours will **not** likely be accurate. This is because though MMS kills the poisons, dead parasites and other material remain in the blood for some time longer. The standard time frame before testing with a microscope to see if one is malaria free, would be to wait a full 24 hours after the person's last dose to be certain that the malaria is gone.

Weaker than Normal Strains of Malaria—When to Reduce the Drops from the Standard 18-drop Dose

➤ If after several malaria victims have taken 18-drop doses and they appear to get sicker at first, this indicates that the type of malaria in the area is a weaker strain and you can give less drops to start with. In this case, the next malaria victim in line can take fewer drops. Reduce the drops by 25% from the standard 18-drop dose. This means you would start giving 13-drop doses of MMS1. If this starts helping people improve or they are not feeling sicker two hours after taking the first dose, then always give a second 13-drop dose (after two hours) just to make totally sure the malaria is gone.

➤ I mentioned earlier that I have been in areas of the world where malaria was handled with a 6-drop dose of MMS1. The general rule of thumb and basic principle of MMS is, if the victim is getting sicker than his sickness is already making him with the MMS1 doses, then you must lower the dose, but **do not stop giving MMS1.** So, in the event that the 13-drop dose is still making one sick, then lower the dose again. Try an 8-drop dose next time, or for the next person, continue the process until you find the comfortable dose that helps the people in that region get well, and does not make them sicker. In this case, generally speaking, we are talking about giving the next person in line a smaller dose.

Note: *Remember, if the first dose was too much or the first 2 doses were too much and it made the malaria victim sicker in any way, then back off and do nothing for several hours as the person will probably be OK as soon as his body eliminates most of the poisons. Give him water to drink until he is feeling better, but never force water on him.*

Stronger than Normal Strains of Malaria—When to Increase the Drops from the Standard 18-drop Dose of MMS1

➤ In the case where a person needs three 18-drop doses to recover from malaria, you can be pretty sure if you are continuing to help people recover their health in that same area, that the next people who come to you from that area will need a stronger first dose than 18 drops. If you have a few people needing three 18-drop doses, this is an indicator that it is time to increase the amount of drops in dosing people if you want to handle malaria in one dose, followed by the suggested second dose to be sure. (In many malaria areas people are unable to hang around for several hours to take their doses. Often there is a small window of time to help them. If the malaria can be knocked out quicker, with less dosing, all the better.) In this case I would increase MMS1 to 25 drops for the first dose, (a little more than 25% because it's a stronger strain of malaria), followed by a second 25-drop dose in two hours.

➤ In the case where an 18-drop dose is not having a sufficient effect and people are not getting well after 3 doses (for several malaria victims), start increasing until you find what works. First try 25-drop doses and then go up to 30 if needed. It may take up to 30 drops to kill the malaria in some areas.

Note: *Once you have established a proper dosage for the area you are in, using water to mix your doses, it is acceptable to use soda or a compatible juice with MMS1 (see pages 42-45 for more information) for the doses because many people have problems with the taste. Then if it should turn out for any reason that the soda or juice doesn't work, in other words, people are no longer getting well, you can always go back to water. One never is really sure that the soda or juice in any given area will not destroy MMS1 (see pages 42-45).*

Children

The standard dosage for helping children recover from malaria must be determined by the weight of the child. Other than this, all the same principles apply as stated above. In other words if you are giving a child the "normal" dosage of MMS1 for malaria and he/she is either getting sicker or not getting well after 3 doses, then you would follow the same procedure as outlined above to decrease or increase the drops. The chart on page 190 will help determine the dosage for children according to weight.

Additional MMS Doses: In all cases if the malaria doses given above do not work and the child is still sick there is a high probability of there being a second disease present in the victim. In that case those who still have sickness present should begin the Starting Procedure, followed by Protocol 1000 as per the instructions for children on pages 256-258.

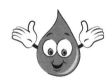

Alzheimer's: After my mother was diagnosed with Alzheimer's she hated the effects of the pill so much that she was willing to try MMS. Her symptoms disappeared almost overnight. The next morning after only drinking 6 drops 3 times she told me the story of how she met my father some 60 years before which was impossible the day before. She continued taking it for a week and then felt so good she stopped taking it. Within one month the symptoms returned. After taking MMS again the symptoms went away again. She had to take a daily maintenance dose to keep it at bay. Thank you Jim Humble you are my Hero. —Keith P., United States

Note: *All the drops on the following chart are referring to activated drops of MMS (MMS1).*

	Malaria Protocol for Children				
	MMS1 Drops Required				
Weight	Minimum Strength Malaria	Low Strength Malaria	Normal Strength Malaria	Stronger Strength Malaria	Maximum Strength Malaria
Babies under 12 lbs (5.5 kg)	1-drop dose	2-drop dose	2-drop dose	3-drop dose	3-drop dose
12-24 lbs (5.5 -11 kg)	3-drop dose	3-drop dose	4-drop dose	5-drop dose	7-drop dose
25-49 lbs (11-23 kg)	4-drop dose	5-drop dose	6-drop dose	8-drop dose	9-drop dose
50-74 lbs. (23-34 kg)	6-drop dose	8-drop dose	10-drop dose	13-drop dose	15-drop dose
75-100 lbs (34-45 kg)	8-drop dose	11-drop dose	14-drop dose	18-drop dose	22-drop dose
100 lbs (45 kg) and Up	10-drop dose	13-drop dose	18-drop dose	23-drop dose	29-drop dose

Chikungunya and Dengue Fever Protocol

Both chikungunya and dengue fever are viral diseases caused by mosquitoes. They are showing up more and more around the world. It is claimed that both diseases have no specific medical treatment. The body can eventually overcome these diseases, however, sometimes after prolonged suffering and/or with difficult complications. Both diseases can cause death. MMS is effective in helping people recover their health in a short time from both chikungunya and dengue fever.

Chikungunya: Generally this disease starts with an abrupt onset of fever, often accompanied by joint pain. Other common symptoms include muscle pain, headache, nausea, fatigue and rash. It can also affect the eyes, ears, and digestion. It is similar to dengue in some ways and can be misdiagnosed in areas where dengue is common. The body generally heals itself from the disease in several weeks, but it is possible for this disease to become chronic and thus last for months or years. Normally, chikungunya shows up somewhere between four to twelve days after being bitten by a mosquito carrying the virus.

Dengue: This disease usually comes on with a fever. It is similar to chikungunya but there are some important differences. There are the extreme muscle and joint pains, and generally a rash, and often pain behind the eyes. It may seem to go away in four or five days or more, but then after two to four days it comes back with a rash that completely covers the body except for the face. The rash will also often be in the palms of the hands and bottoms of the feet. It may go away in a few days or it might last much longer. There can also be chills during this disease. It sometimes gets very severe and can cause hemorrhaging and death, especially in small children. Dengue fever shows up sometime within three to fifteen days after being bitten by the mosquito carrying the dengue virus.

Both dengue fever and chikungunya can be overcome by MMS1 or MMS2 which kills the virus and then the body can quickly rebuild health. Overcoming these diseases is not the same as with malaria. Malaria is a parasite which is a much larger microorganism and requires an initial large shock (dose) of MMS1 to eradicate. Viruses require the presence of MMS 1 or 2 over a period of time to destroy them. We have had the best success with these two diseases by starting them off with two stronger than normal doses of MMS1, then going right in to Protocol 1000, which keeps MMS1 present in the body for eight hours or a little longer each day. MMS2 can be substituted for MMS1 (when not available) in this protocol, as per the directions below.

Instructions—Using MMS1 for Dengue and Chikungunya

Step 1

❑ Do Protocol 6 and 6, which is taking a 6-drop dose of MMS1, then wait an hour and take a second 6-drop MMS1 dose. (See page 169 for full instructions on Protocol 6 and 6.)

Note: *If the first 6-drop dose causes nausea, drop to 1/2 of that (a 3-drop dose), for the second dose.*

Step 2

❑ After two 6-drop doses, (or the 6-drop/3-drop dose if you had to cut back) continue Protocol 1000 as per the instructions on page 84. Continue Protocol 1000 for at least three weeks (21 days).

Children

➤ If you are helping a child please follow the proper dosages for children for Protocol 6 and 6 and Protocol 1000. Remember, dosing for children is determined according to the child's weight. See Chapter 13 for instructions on how to adjust protocol dosages for children. Follow all rules; for example, lower the dosage when nausea or increased sickness shows up.

Instructions—Using MMS2 for Dengue and Chikungunya

If MMS1 is not available, but MMS2 (calcium hypochlorite) is, you can substitute MMS2 for MMS1 for dengue and chikungunya. Carefully follow the steps below:

Step 1

❑ First, thoroughly read the instructions in the section on MMS2 Details, page 274, regarding MMS2. Do not use MMS2 without having a clear understanding of how it works.

Step 2

❑ Once you have an understanding of MMS2 and you are fully aware of the needed precautions for using it, make up your gel or vegetable capsules. Use either #0 or #1 size capsules, according to the instructions on pages 275-278.

❑ Please note that you need to fill the capsules with a small quantity of MMS2 at first and work up to the recommended amount. This protocol calls for taking 5 doses (5 capsules in total, 1 capsule per dose) of MMS2 a day. On the first day start with the lowest amount to fill the capsules for the first 2 doses, then begin filling the capsules with more MMS2 in increments, according to instructions on page 276, Step 3. If you experience sickness, more than what you are already experiencing from the illness, then cut back on the amount of MMS2 and go at a slower pace to build up to the recommended amount of MMS2 in each capsule. Follow the Three Golden Rules of MMS.

Step 3

❑ Take 1 MMS2 capsule every two hours until you have taken 5 capsules in a day.

❑ Continue taking 5 capsules a day until the sickness is gone. Generally dengue and chikungunya will be gone in three or four days, but nevertheless continue with this protocol. Do not stop for a full three weeks. This is to insure you are totally over the illness and for prevention against relapse.

Children

I do not recommend MMS2 for small children, nor for all children no matter what their age or weight. There are exceptions to this, but do not proceed giving children MMS2 until you read the guidelines and instructions regarding **MMS2 and children** on pages 259-260. If after reading that you determine the child can take MMS2 capsules, proceed as per the following instructions.

❑ Use size #3 vegetable or gel capsules for children, filled 1/8 full with MMS2 to start and work up to filling it 3/4 full.

❑ If nausea or increased sickness shows up, reduce the powder in the capsules by one half. If needed, keep reducing until the capsules do not cause **additional** sickness or nausea. You can try again to slowly increase the powder to the recommended dosage, but cut back any time additional sickness occurs.

❑ Remember, **only give this to a child who is old enough and can be trusted** to properly swallow a capsule without breaking it open in the process.

Ebola Virus

Ebola virus disease is severe and often fatal. At the time of this writing, it reportedly kills up to 50% of people who are infected. It spreads mostly by contact with a person who is infected and sometimes through contact with a surface such as a desk, chair, or table with which an infected person has made contact. Symptoms may include fever, nausea, vomiting, diarrhea, red eyes, raised rashes, chest pain, coughing, stomach pain, weight loss, bleeding from the eyes, ears, nose, rectum and much internal bleeding.

In West Africa, Genesis II Church Health Ministers have had success in helping people overcome Ebola virus disease. This was confirmed, when possible, in lab tests before and after in some of the cases.

The protocol that was used was basically the same as the Chikungunya/Dengue Fever Protocol (see page 190). Victims recovered their health in seven to ten days. I strongly suggest however, that even if feeling well in a week to ten days, that one complete the full 21 days of the protocol in order to avoid a possible relapse.

Zika Virus

At the time of writing this book the Zika virus, also spread by a mosquito with similarities to both chikungunya and dengue fever, is becoming more prevalent in the world. Currently, according to the CDC (Centers for Disease Control and Prevention), most people infected with Zika virus disease will not have symptoms. The incubation period for Zika virus disease is not known, but it is likely to be a few days to a week. The most common symptoms of Zika are fever, rash, joint pain, or conjunctivitis (red eyes), muscle pain and headache.

To date, we have not received sufficient on-going proof of success using MMS1 or MMS2 with the Zika virus. However, we have received confirmation from some of our Health Ministers, of people recovering full health from Zika after following the protocol outlined in this book for chikungunya and dengue fever.

If you are in a Zika area and suspect you have been infected, or desire to help others who are infected, I would suggest this same protocol. Keep up hourly doses as given in the protocol until the symptoms are totally gone and health is restored.

Mosquito Bites

When bitten by a mosquito, dab one drop of unactivated MMS right on the bite and gently rub it in. The itching should stop in several minutes. It is not usually necessary to wash the MMS off after rubbing it in, but if you prefer, wash the area with soap and water after waiting at least five minutes.

MRSA Protocol

MRSA (Methicillin-resistant Staphylococcus Aureus), is commonly known as *staph.* Both on the inside and the outside of the body this infection can become quite a problem. It is an infection that is resistant to all known antibiotics. Sadly, every year MRSA kills many people. Fortunately with MMS, it is easy to control.

Many with MRSA have recovered by taking MMS1 protocols, beginning with the Starting Procedure and then on to Protocol 1000, and continuing on with more protocols if needed as outlined in this book. Those with skin eruptions may want to try using chlorine dioxide gas (as explained in the following instructions) on these external eruptions, as this handles the infection quite easily. This same procedure is also effective for any standard boil.

Instructions for Overcoming MRSA (and Boils)

Step 1

❑ Begin by taking MMS1 with the Starting Procedure, followed by Protocol 1000 (see pages 79-87).

Note: *For those who have MRSA that is manifesting on the outside of the body, or those who have a boil, immediately begin the following steps using chlorine dioxide gas, while simultaneously beginning Step 1 above. If preferred, the MMS1/DMSO Patch Protocol can also be used on MRSA sores or boils in place of the following procedure (see page 135).*

Step 2

❑ Find a glass, cup or bowl that will fit over the MRSA infection or the boil. It is best if the bowl or cup is clear glass so you can see through it and observe what is happening. Glass is preferable, but a clear plastic container would work. If you can't find this, then use a regular coffee cup or bowl.

Step 3

❑ Clear the area around the MRSA infection or boil so that the cup or glass can sit securely over and around the infection and so that no MMS gas will be able to escape. You will be holding the glass in place. It will not be there longer than five minutes.

Step 4

❑ Determine how many drops of MMS1 (activated MMS)
to use. Depending on the size of the infection, use from
5 to 20 drops of MMS1 (using 4% HCl or 50% citric
acid to activate). Use 5 drops for a MRSA infection or
a boil about 1/2 inch (1.25 cm) in diameter. Use 10
drops of MMS1 for a MRSA infection or boil 1 inch (2.5
cm) across. For any sore 2 inches (5 cm) or larger in
diameter, use 15 to 20 drops.

Step 5

❑ Using Step 4 above as your guide to the number of
drops to use, put these drops in your container and
immediately cover the infection or boil. Be careful to
hold the container so that the MMS1 will not run down
on your skin, and so you are not allowing any gas to
escape. You may have to lie down or lean over,
depending on the location of the boil.

❑ **Do not apply this for longer than five minutes
maximum**, to avoid burning the skin. If one has
particularly sensitive skin, it would be best to do this
procedure for only three minutes the first time in order
to see how the skin reacts. If the skin reacts well, it
can be repeated again in four hours (see directions
below), and for up to five minutes the second time if
needed. But remember, **no longer than five minutes**.

Step 6

❑ The chlorine dioxide gas generated by the activated
MMS will cover the infection in seconds, and you will
be able to see the infection open up, and the inside of
the infection will drain out in a couple of minutes.
Stand, or sit, or lie down so that the infection—be it on

the side of your arm, or face, or leg—can drain, allowing the pus to drain downward into your container.

❑ Have some tissues on hand to absorb the remaining pus when you remove the container.

Step 7

❑ After doing Steps 1 through 6 one time, cover the area with Vaseline, which will help prevent any further infection.

Step 8

❑ If it appears that some pus may still be remaining in the infection, you may repeat Steps 1 through 6 a second time. Do this **only after you wait at least four hours after the first application**, and **only after you have washed off the Vaseline** as thoroughly as possible with soap and water.

❑ After repeating Steps 1 through 6 a second time, once more cover the area with Vaseline to prevent infection.

Step 9

❑ You may repeat Steps 1 thru 6 a third time, but again, **only after you wait at least four hours after the second application**, and **only after you have washed off the Vaseline** as thoroughly as possible with soap and water.

Step 10

❑ In a rare case where pain and soreness persists, you may repeat Steps 1 through 6 once every four hours until the condition clears. At this point, wait four hours between each application of Steps 1 through 6. Each

time you repeat Steps 1 through 6, you should coat
the area with Vaseline to prevent further infection and
be sure to wash off the Vaseline before further
applications of Step 1 through 6.

Step 11

❑ Most likely, there will be a hole in the skin and flesh
where the infection was located. You may put a little
Vaseline in the hole. It should heal up in two or three
days. The Vaseline prevents further re-infection. You
may spray it with the MMS1 spray bottle (see
instructions on page 76), but that is seldom needed.

Step 12

❑ As per Step 1 above, the person with MRSA should
complete the Starting Procedure, followed by Protocol
1000. If they are also using MMS1 on skin sores, and
the sores clear up before the 3-week period that
Protocol 1000 calls for is finished, it would nevertheless
be best to finish the 21 days of Protocol 1000. This will
further cleanse the body of unwanted bacteria and
toxins.

Daily MMS1 Maintenance Dose

A daily maintenance dose of MMS is very important.
With the tremendous amount of toxins, poisons and other
health hazards that cause disease in today's society,
prevention is essential to help one enjoy a healthy and
balanced life. MMS1 can help you reach this goal. A good
time to take your maintenance dose is before bedtime,
which aids the detoxification process during sleep. In
times of stress or when local sickness is "going around"
flu, coughs, colds, etc., or anytime you have extra exposure to toxins, such as during travels, and so on, I suggest
doubling the maintenance dose. That is, if you take a daily

maintenance dose and you have extra exposure, take it twice a day (morning and evening) instead of once. If you take a maintenance dose 3 times a week, instead take it daily during these times.

You will notice on the dosage charts below I am suggesting that adults under 60 years of age take a maintenance dose 3 times a week, and yet I suggest children take a daily maintenance dose (adjusted according to their weight). This is because children, as a rule, are exposed to a wide variety of toxins throughout the day; they play on the floor or in the dirt, put dirty hands into their mouths, etc.

Daily Maintenace Dose—Children	
Age and Weight	**Daily Dosage**
12 lbs or less (5.5 kg or less)	1 drop daily
12-24 lbs (5.5-11 kg)	2 drops daily
25-49 lbs (11-23 kg)	3 drops daily
50-74 lbs (23-34 kg)	4 drops daily
75-100 lbs (34-45 kg)	5 drops daily
100-lbs and up (45 kg and up)	6 drops daily

Daily Maintenance Dose—Adults	
Age and Weight	**Daily Dosage**
Adults 60 years and over, 100 to 200 lbs	6 drops daily
Adults 60 years and over, 200 lbs and over	8 drops daily
Adults 60 years and under, 100 to 200 lbs	6 drops 3x a week
Adults 60 years and under, 200 lbs and over	8 drops 3x a week

Note: If you need to use MMS2 for your daily maintenance dose, please see Protocol 4000 notes, on page 172 for instructions.

Morgellans and MMS: I tell you it was a miracle how I got MMS in my hands. I was suffering with what I believe now to be Morgellons. My doctor told me, "I can't diagnose it and I can't treat it" and walked out of the room. I also had been fighting Candida for years with nothing working, it would get better and come back. My daughter had asked me to find a product that had helped her with a health issue. I found a product I thought was what she wanted. Soon I received an email saying my MMS was being shipped. I researched MMS. I could not believe what I was seeing, it was exactly what I needed for the symptoms I was having. I started the protocol and almost immediately the sores and itching were getting better.

Today the Morgellons and Candida are gone. I have gone to iridologist and when she saw me she said. "My goodness I have never seen anyone heal like that, what did you do?" I told her how I got the MMS. She said you need to write that down and share it with others who may be suffering with Morgellons. I am alive and healthy today because of MMS. I was contemplating suicide because of the pain and itching and the inability to sleep for a year prior to finding this wonderful product. I believe God let me stumble onto an inexpensive product that would heal my body. Thank you Jim Humble. —Joy S., United States

Edema Gone: I had a bad case of edema on my legs and thought I had a blood clot. I treated myself with Protocol 1000 and within a few days - my legs were back to normal. No pitting, swelling, etc. —C.P., United States

Chapter 12

Emergency Protocols

The basic idea when an emergency strikes is to act fast. You want to get something into the body that will help handle the condition and kill the poisons that might be present. Below, you will find some emergency situations that we have found MMS to be particularly helpful in. This is, by all means, not meant to be a comprehensive list. MMS will also work for many other emergency situations. Keep in mind with these protocols one may need to disregard the advice given elsewhere in this book of not taking too much MMS, while at the same time, being careful not to go too far. If you so choose, follow these instructions and listen to what the body tells you—be it your body or someone else's.

Disclaimer

These Emergency Protocols are an alternative for those individuals who find themselves in a dire situation and unable to seek mainstream medical help for one reason or another, be it logistics, financial, or otherwise, such as a personal decision to not want to go to the hospital and subject oneself to allopathic procedures. The decision to choose an alternative is a personal choice. The responsibility is 100% on each and every individual for any and all use made of any information herein. If one is not prepared to take full responsibility for their own health, be it in a severe or less severe case, I strongly advise they seek conventional medical attention.

Stings and Bites

Stinging or biting insects, scorpions, or spiders can be hazardous to one's health. The results of stings or bites from these critters range from being irritating, to serious, to possibly fatal if not treated. The decision to follow the information outlined below is up to the individual. In any given situation, each person must decide what to do.

For those who are allergic to bee stings and other stings that are poisonous, it has been my personal experience that MMS has been effective in handling the condition, while eliminating the risk of serious side-effects of pharmaceuticals. For example, both spider bite and scorpion antivenin almost always list several adverse side effects, including the possibility of death. MMS, as far as we know, has never caused permanent side effects to anyone. The following procedures for bites and stings have worked for many people, however, there is no 100% guarantee.

Scorpion Stings

Most scorpion stings are not deadly, they are just painful. You cannot however, depend on the idea that the one that just stung you is not deadly. There is one species of scorpion in the US that is deadly. There are over 2,000 species of scorpions throughout the world with only a few being of the deadly species, but again, never assume that the one that just stung you is not a deadly scorpion. If stung by a scorpion, I would try the following steps. If I was not getting better in a reasonable amount of time, and seemed to be getting worse, I would go to a hospital or clinic that has antivenin serum. Pray that the antivenin has no negative effect as the same problem exists for scorpion stings as spider bites, in that death is one of the possible side effects often listed for the antivenin.

Immediately After Being Stung by a Scorpion

Step 1

❏ In the event of a scorpion sting, start taking MMS1 by mouth immediately. Take one 6-drop dose of MMS1 in 1/2 cup (4 ounces/120 ml) of water, followed by a second 6-drop dose of MMS1, one-half hour later.

Note: *This is similar to Protocol 6 and 6 (see page 169), however in this case the doses are taken closer together, one-half hour apart, instead of one hour apart. In the event of following this procedure for a child, follow the same dosage rules as Protocol 6 and 6, adjusting the dose according to weight as per the chart on page 265.*

❏ If the first MMS1 dose makes you nauseous or causes you to vomit, drink more water (8 ounces) and try to vomit again if you can. In this case vomiting is good and will help expel the poison.

Step 2

Simultaneously with Step 1, immediately after you have taken your first oral dose of MMS1—begin to neutralize the sting poison:

❏ In a clean, dry glass, activate 3 drops of MMS with 3 drops of acid activator. Count 30 seconds. **Do not add water.**

❏ Dip the end of your finger into the MMS1 mixture and dab it on the site of the sting. (Try to get it directly on the point where the scorpion attacked and not too much on the surrounding skin.) Try to apply pressure to force the MMS1 down into the hole. Do this every five minutes or so. Rinse your finger after every application.

❑ Mix up a fresh dose of MMS1 as per the instructions above, every 15 to 20 minutes.

❑ Stop applying the MMS1 mixture directly on the sting once the pain of the sting is gone.

❑ Continue for a longer period of time if the sting continues to hurt or itch.

Note: *Stop using the MMS1 for several hours if the skin begins to get badly irritated around the sting.*

Step 3

❑ After taking the second 6-drop dose of MMS1, continue taking a 3-drop dose of MMS1 every waking hour, until all negative symptoms subside. Do this even if it takes a few days.

Note: *A 3-drop dose is the standard Protocol 1000 dose. In the case where a child is stung by a scorpion, follow the dosage guide as per weight for Protocol 1000 for children (see page 258).*

Bee and Wasp Stings

For many people bee and wasp stings do not pose a big problem and cause little trouble. There are some home remedies that are effective for these stings, such as making a baking soda paste for a bee sting, or using vinegar for a wasp sting. Just the same, if you have a minor reaction to a sting this protocol can help. If you are **allergic** to bee or wasp stings and have a serious reaction to them, I suggest you go directly to this protocol.

The bee sting is **acidic** in nature and can be neutralized with unactivated MMS (sodium chlorite 22.4% solution in water), this is without mixing it with an acid activator. The wasp sting is **alkaline** and it must be neutralized with acid. You can use either 4% HCl acid or 50% citric acid. Following are instructions for neutralizing the poison at the site of a bee or wasp sting.

Instructions for Bee and Wasp Stings

Step 1

❑ In the event of a bee or wasp sting, start taking MMS1 by mouth immediately. Take one 6-drop dose of MMS1 in 1/2 cup (4 ounces/120 ml) of water, followed by a second 6-drop dose of MMS1, one-half hour later.

Note: *This is similar to Protocol 6 and 6 (see page 169), however in this case the doses are taken closer together, one-half hour apart, instead of one hour apart. In the event of following this procedure for a child, follow the same dosage rules as Protocol 6 and 6, adjusting the dose according to weight as per the chart on page 265.*

❑ If the first MMS1 dose makes you nauseous or causes you to vomit, drink more water (8 ounces) and try to vomit again if you can. In this case vomiting is good and will help expel the poison.

Step 2

❑ Simultaneously with Step 1, immediately after you have taken your first oral dose of MMS1—begin to neutralize the sting poison. Please note that these **instructions for Step 2 are different for the bee and the wasp sting.**

Bee Sting

❑ **Use MMS (sodium chlorite, 22.4%** in purified water) but without activating it. The unactivated MMS is highly alkaline and it neutralizes the acid of the bee sting.

❑ Put 4 or 5 drops of MMS in a clean dry glass. **Do not add water**.

❑ Dip the end of your finger into the unactivated MMS and carefully rub it on the sting. Press hard to force a tiny amount into the sting. Repeat this every five minutes or so.

❑ Stop applying the sodium chlorite (MMS unactivated) directly on the sting once the pain of the sting is gone.

❑ Continue for a longer period of time, up to an hour, if the sting continues to hurt or itch.

❑ After you have stopped applying the MMS, rinse the area thoroughly with clean water.

If the Sting Continues to Hurt After One Hour

❑ Rinse the area thoroughly with clean water.

❑ After applying **only MMS** (unactivated MMS) for one hour, the acidic nature of the bee sting is sufficiently neutralized. If it still hurts, you can now apply activated MMS (MMS1) to destroy any poison that may be left. Activate 3 drops of MMS (sodium chlorite) with 3 drops of activator acid and count 30 seconds. **Do not add water**.

❑ Dab it on the sting and carefully rub it in.

❑ This can be repeated every five minutes or so for up to half an hour.

Wasp Sting

❑ **Do not use MMS. Use the activator acid alone,** (4% HCl or 50% citric acid). If these are not available, straight lemon juice or vinegar is the next best thing.

❑ Put 4 or 5 drops of acid in a clean dry glass. **Do not add water**.

❑ Dip the end of your finger into the acid and dab it on the site of the sting. (Try to get it directly on the sting site and not too much on the surrounding skin.) Carefully rub it into the sting hole, but press hard to get some acid into the hole to neutralize the sting poison.

❑ Do this every five minutes or so. Rinse your finger after every application.

❑ Stop applying the acid directly on the sting once the pain of the sting is gone.

❑ Continue for a longer period of time, up to an hour, if the sting continues to hurt or itch.

❑ After you have stopped applying the acid, rinse the area thoroughly with clean water.

If the Sting Continues to Hurt After One Hour

❑ Rinse the area thoroughly with clean water.

❑ After applying **only acid** to the wasp sting for one hour, the alkaline nature of the sting should be neutralized. If it still hurts, you can now apply activated MMS (MMS1) to destroy any of the remaining poison. Activate 3 drops of MMS (sodium chlorite) with 3 drops of activator acid and count 30 seconds. **Do not add water**.

❑ Dab it on the sting and carefully rub it in.

❑ This can be repeated every five minutes or so for up to half an hour.

Step 3

❑ After the second 6-drop dose of MMS1, continue taking a 3-drop dose of MMS1 every waking hour, until all negative symptoms subside. Do this even if it takes a few days.

Note: *A 3-drop dose is the standard Protocol 1000 dose. In the case where a child is stung by a bee or wasp, follow the dosage guide as per weight for Protocol 1000 for children (see page 258).*

Spider Bites

Both Black Widow and Brown Recluse spiders are not only painful, but they are deadly. I have listed them separately, each with a distinct protocol. If you suspect your bite is a Black Widow or a Brown Recluse, please refer to the specific protocol respectively, as these protocols have been known to work (so far) every time. (See pages 213, 217.)

If you suspect some other poisonous spider has bitten you (there are many poisonous spiders throughout the world), the following simple remedy may be effective. If this remedy does not overcome the pain and swelling within a reasonable amount of time (a couple of hours), I suggest going to a hospital or a clinic that has antivenin.

Note: *MMS is an oxidizer and has been known to oxidize and destroy many kinds of poison. However, there is no way that we could test the ability of MMS to destroy literally hundreds of types of spider poison that exist. It is our experience that MMS will help with most poison situations, but the decision to use or not use MMS in the case of a spider bite is the complete responsibility of the individual.*

Immediately After Being Bitten by a Poisonous Spider

Step 1

❑ Read the introductory paragraphs in both the Black Widow (page 217) and the Brown Recluse (page 213) Spider Protocols , to make sure the bite wasn't one of those.

❑ In the event of a spider bite, start taking MMS1 by mouth immediately. Take one 6-drop dose of MMS1 in 1/2 cup (4 ounces/120 ml) of water, followed by a second 6-drop dose of MMS1, one-half hour later.

Note: *This is similar to Protocol 6 and 6 (see page 169), however in this case the doses are taken closer together, one-half hour apart, instead of one hour apart. In the event of following this procedure for a child, follow the same dosage rules as Protocol 6 and 6, adjusting the dose according to weight as per the chart on page 265.*

❑ If the first MMS1 dose makes you nauseous or causes you to vomit, drink more water (8 ounces) and try to vomit again if you can. In this case vomiting is good and will help expel the poison.

Step 2

❏ Simultaneously with Step 1, immediately after you have taken your first oral dose of MMS1—begin to neutralize the bite poison.

❏ In a clean, dry glass, activate 3 drops of MMS with 3 drops of acid activator. Count 30 seconds. **Do not add water.**

❏ Dip the end of your finger into the MMS1 mixture and dab it on the bite. (Try to get it directly on the bite and not too much on the surrounding skin.) Do this every five minutes or so. Rinse your finger after every application.

❏ Mix up a fresh dose of MMS1 as per the instructions above, every 15 to 20 minutes.

❏ Stop applying the MMS1 mixture directly on the bite once the pain of the bite is gone.

❏ Continue for a longer period of time if the bite continues to hurt or itch.

Note: *Stop using the MMS1 for several hours if the skin begins to get badly irritated around the bite.*

Step 3

❏ After taking the second 6-drop dose of MMS1, continue taking a 3-drop dose of MMS1 every waking hour, until all negative symptoms subside. Do this even if it takes a few days.

Note: *A 3-drop dose is the standard Protocol 1000 dose. In the case where a child is bitten by a poisonous spider,* *follow the dosage guide as per weight for Protocol 1000 for children (see page 258).*

Brown Recluse Protocol

Overall, the Brown Recluse spider is considered the most dangerous spider bite that anyone might receive (outside of rare species in the jungle). Many people have died from Brown Recluse bites. One website lists that each year 25% of people bitten die from the bite. This may or may not be true; however, there is no doubt that such a bite can give a person a great deal of trouble. I have yet to meet a medical doctor who can offer a successful treatment for a Brown Recluse bite. However, I have found the procedure below to be quite effective. With the Brown Recluse, you want to be sure to tend to any bite as soon as possible.

Note: *I lived for 40 years in the deserts of California and Nevada, during which time I personally treated 20 to 25 people for Brown Recluse bites with the zinc oxide salve mentioned below. In the last several years I also added MMS. The zinc oxide salve always worked with or without MMS. The decision to use or not use this protocol is totally your responsibility. In my opinion this protocol can save your life as the medical system has no effective treatment for the Brown Recluse spider bite.*

How do You Know if You Have a Brown Recluse Bite?

Normally, you will not know right off that you've been bitten by a Brown Recluse, unless you actually see the spider bite you. With a Brown Recluse, you never feel the bite. But if you have been bitten, usually after about four hours, you will begin to feel itching. It won't feel very strong at first, not even enough to scratch, but then it will become more intense. When you look at the area that itches, you will notice a small red spot about the size of a grain of wheat, and by that time it is likely you will have scratched it several times. From that point things worsen fairly rapidly. The itching becomes extremely bad and then turns into painful itching, and this then becomes acute pain. The time it takes to get to this point of acute pain can vary, usually anywhere from 8 to 24 hours.

If nothing is done, the pain will get worse until you go to the doctor where medicine is prescribed for the pain. The pain killer may possibly take away the pain, but it doesn't address the underlying cause of the pain. Soon a tiny hole begins to develop. The hole can get bigger and bigger and will eventually go all the way to the bone. Depending on where the bite is, people have been known to lose half of a leg, or most of their face as the hole gets bigger. In severe cases, some people suffer up to two years before they die. I am sharing these details, in hopes that you can avoid this situation, and likewise help someone else if necessary.

Instructions for Brown Recluse Spider Bite

Step 1

❑ Begin a slight variation of Protocol 6 and 6 (see page 169). Take a 6-drop dose of MMS1, then take the second 6-drop dose after only one-half hour as opposed to one hour.

❑ One-half hour after taking the second 6-drop dose begin Protocol 1000. But begin by taking a 1/2-drop dose the first hour and increase the amount each hour by 1/2 drop, building up to a 3-drop dose each hour. Continue with Protocol 1000 for two weeks, and if needed for a third week, or as long as necessary.

Step 2

❑ Simultaneously right after the first MMS1 dose, begin applying zinc oxide. Mix equal parts of zinc oxide and Vaseline Petroleum Jelly. Make this into a paste.

Step 3

❑ Spread a generous portion of the salve on the bite area and gently rub it in for a minute or two.

❑ Then after a minute or two, add more salve to the bite area to make sure it is nice and thick. Cover the area with gauze and adhesive tape. Bandage it well, but not so tight that it does not get some air.

Step 4

❑ Repeat Step 3 (above) after four hours. It is not necessary to wash off the former application.

Step 5

❑ Repeat Step 3 (above) again, after another four hours. This will be the third application of the zinc oxide salve.

Step 6

❑ After three applications of the zinc oxide ointment, (each one four hours apart) the pain and itching should subside. If however, there is still discomfort, begin using the MMS1 spray bottle, which is a solution of 10 activated drops of MMS to 1 ounce of purified water, (see page 76). Wash the area before using the spray bottle.

❑ Spray the affected area every 20 minutes or so, until everything is all cleared up.

Notes

➤   Remember, throughout this procedure the victim should be taking MMS1 as per Protocol 1000, every hour on the hour for eight consecutive hours a day. Continue for two weeks, or longer if needed.

➤   In the event that you cannot get zinc oxide, you might be able to find zinc chloride which can be used instead. Zinc chloride or oxide will usually produce results in less than four hours, but if you have any continued problem at all from using zinc chloride, try your best to get some zinc oxide and repeat the procedure again.

➤   There are various brands of Petroleum Jelly on the market. I recommend the original "Vaseline" brand for mixing with clay or zinc oxide to make a salve. Vaseline (the original, which is triple-purified to be 100% pure) has the unique ability to wet and penetrate and remain in place on the skin for hours longer than most oils. Sometimes coconut oil, olive oil and other oils can be used to carry various medicinal substances to the skin and hold them there. However, nothing matches the ability of Vaseline to hold healing substances in contact with the skin for hours while at the same time act as a healing agent itself. Use the various other oils only if you cannot obtain the Vaseline.

➤   The procedure above with zinc oxide has been known to relieve a Brown Recluse spider bite within four hours.

Variation: If available in your country, *Desitin* Baby Diaper Rash Ointment—Extra Strength, has also been successful in healing Brown Recluse Spider bites. This formula contains zinc oxide. Check the ingredients to be sure you get the one that contains 40% zinc oxide, which is the Extra Strength Formula. The formulas that contain

20 to 25% zinc oxide may work, but the 40% formula is more certain to work.

Black Widow Protocol

It is not a fable; the Black Widow indeed has a bright red hourglass shape on her belly. Many people are bitten by the Black Widow spider yearly, but very few die from her bite. Probably less than 5 people die in the US each year according to most websites.

Note: *I lived for 40 years in the deserts of California and Nevada, during which time I personally helped more than 20 people bitten by a Black Widow spider with the protocol given below. It always worked. In addition, I was bitten by a Black Widow spider twice, and it worked for me. The use of Aloe vera in this protocol is something I found in an old book of remedies when I was a young fellow about 20 years of age. So people have been using this part of the protocol to handle Black Widow bites for many years! I have since added MMS1, and have found the combination of the two to bring good results. The decision to follow this procedure however, is totally your responsibility.*

The bite of the Black Widow is different than the Brown Recluse spider. Normally with this bite there is immediate pain, followed by a number of possible reactions. There can be muscle cramps, abdominal pain (stomach ache), weakness, tremors, body aching, and in more severe cases, nausea, vomiting, fainting, dizziness, chest pain and difficulty breathing.

For the Black Widow bite, there is an antivenin available. I am not telling you one way or the other to take the antivenin. I didn't use it myself when I was bitten by a Black Widow, but many have used it. However, like most pharmaceutical drugs, there is a long list of side effects from this drug, including possible death for those who have a history of asthma. Other reactions include rash, hives, itching, difficulty breathing, difficulty swallowing, tightness in the chest, and swelling of the mouth, face, lips and tongue. An alternative to taking the antivenin if you so choose, is MMS1 and *Aloe vera*.

Instructions for Black Widow Bite

Step 1

❑ The first thing to do is to begin a slight variation of Protocol 6 and 6 (see page 169).

❑ Take a 6-drop dose of MMS1, but in the case of a Black Widow bite, take the second 6-drop dose after only one-half hour as opposed to one hour.

Step 2

❑ Simultaneously, immediately after taking the first 6-drop dose of MMS1, as per the step above, and while waiting to take the second 6-drop dose, do the following:

❑ Obtain a large fresh *Aloe vera* leaf.

❑ Cut off the serrated edges and then cut the leaf open lengthwise. Then cut a piece about 2 inches x 2 inches (5 cm x 5 cm) and put the fresh *Aloe vera*—flesh side down—right onto the bite. Hold the piece in place and cover it with gauze and secure it firmly with adhesive tape. Be sure that air cannot get between the *Aloe vera* leaf and the bite on the skin.

❑ In an emergency, use whatever is available to keep the *Aloe vera* in place until you can get the proper supplies, (i.e. gauze/adhesive tape) but secure it down well so there is no air getting to the bite.

❑ Leave this on for 12 hours and the bite should be OK. However, to make sure, repeat this procedure one more time with a fresh piece of *Aloe vera*. Tape it on for another 12 hours and that should be all that is needed.

Step 3

❑ One-half hour after taking the first 6-drop dose, and hopefully applying the *Aloe vera,* take the second 6-drop dose.

Step 4

❑ One-half hour after taking the second 6-drop dose (hopefully you will have applied the first application of *Aloe vera* during this time) begin Protocol 1000. But begin by taking a 1/2-drop dose the first hour and increase the amount each hour by 1/2 drop, building up to a 3-drop dose each hour, as Protocol 1000 calls for.

❑ Follow through with Protocol 1000 for two weeks, taking MMS1, eight consecutive hours a day. If needed, continue for a third week on Protocol 1000, or as long as necessary.

Snake Bite Protocol

This protocol has not been widely used or proven, due to a lack of snake bite cases coming to us. I did have a test case of a rattle snake biting a small dog. With MMS, two days after the bite, the dog was fine. However, the fact is, MMS1 neutralizes poisons of most kinds. The poison of the snake variety is a very complex molecule, and MMS1 (chlorine dioxide) destroys complex molecules by oxidation. So in an emergency, it would be better to do something rather than nothing. And in any case, it would be a good idea to apply this protocol in addition to whatever medical treatment is used, but do not allow anyone to cut into your snake bite because it can make the situation worse.

Instructions—Snake Bite

Caution: With a snake bite you do not want to waste time! It is vital that as quickly as possible you start getting MMS1 into the body as per the dosages given below.

Step 1

❑ Immediately take a 12-drop dose of MMS1.

Step 2

❑ Simultaneously, in conjunction with taking MMS1 doses, apply the Snake Bite Patch on the bite area. Do this immediately after taking the first MMS1 dose as per Step 1 above. Please note, the **snake bite patch is a significantly different formula than the MMS1/DMSO Patch** on page 135 in this book. **Never, ever put DMSO on a snake bite,** as this will take the poison further into the body, not draw it out. See Making a Snake Bite Patch, following Step 6 of this protocol, page 221.

Step 3

❑ One-half hour later, after the first 12-drop dose of MMS1, take a second dose of MMS1, this time, a 6-drop dose.

Step 4

❑ One-half hour later, after the second dose of MMS1, take a third dose. The third dose will be a 6-drop dose of MMS1.

Recap: When someone has been bitten by a snake, they should immediately take a 12-drop dose of MMS1. One-half hour later, they should take a 6-drop dose of MMS1. One-half hour after that, take another 6-drop dose of MMS1. This is 3 MMS1 doses taken one-half hour apart. After the first 12-drop dose of MMS1, they should apply the patch for a snake bite.

Step 5

❑ One-half hour later, (after taking the 3 doses of MMS1 mentioned in Steps 2, 3, and 4 above) begin Protocol 1000. That is, take a 3-drop dose of MMS1 every hour for eight consecutive hours a day. In the case of a snake bite, you can skip the Starting Procedure.

Step 6

❑ Continue Protocol 1000 for at least two weeks, or longer if there is any indication of the snake bite still causing trouble. Reduce the number of hourly drops by one half if there is nausea, diarrhea or ill feelings. Reduce, but do not stop taking them hourly.

Making a Snake Bite Patch as Required in Step 3 Above

Note and Caution: *The recipe for the patch for a snake bite is different than is described in the MMS1/DMSO Patch Protocol on page 135 of this book.* **The patch for a snake bite does not contain DMSO. Do not use DMSO in a patch for a snake bite.** *This can be a serious mistake.*

The DMSO will spread the poison and take it deeper into the tissues, worsening the problem.

Step 1

❑ Activate 10 drops of MMS with 10 drops of 50% citric acid or 4% HCl. Count to 30 seconds, and then add 20 drops of water.

❑ Immediately pour this mixture on a piece of gauze approximately 2 inches by 2 inches (5 cm by 5 cm) and at least two layers thick. If this mixture is not enough to completely soak the patch, then double the recipe. Activate 10 more drops of MMS and add 20 drops water as per the same formula in the point above, so as to be able to soak the patch in the mixture.

❑ In the case of an extra large snake bite, you can adjust the patch to include more than 10 drops of activated MMS. (Please note, the Snake Bite Patch calls for adding 2 drops of water for every 1 drop of activated MMS.)

Step 2

❑ Tape the soaked gauze onto the snake bite, leave it for 15 to 20 minutes—no more!

❑ Remember, the **patch for the snake bite does not contain DMSO.**

Step 3

❑ Apply a fresh patch (a second patch) in one hour. This will mean in the first two hours after being bitten, you will have applied two MMS1 patches. Add more water to the patch if you notice irritation of the skin.

Step 4

❑ After the first two patches, wait three hours and apply another fresh patch, and continue applying a fresh patch every three hours.

Notes

➤ *In total, you should keep applying the patches according to these instructions, every three hours, for a 24 hour period. (Set an alarm during sleep hours and get up to apply the patch.) Remember, you are also doing Protocol 1000 during this time.*

➤ *If the MMS1 patch is burning your skin, continue by adding some more water until the patch is not burning, but do not add more water than necessary.*

Food Poisoning Protocol
(or Any Poison Received by Mouth)

According to the CDC (Centers for Disease Control), over 5,000 people die from food borne poisons or diseases in the United States each year, with similar figures worldwide. The point here being, it is advantageous to know what to do about food poisoning.

A friend of mine was poisoned once while eating dinner with myself and others. He got up from the table and immediately collapsed and fell to the floor. I helped him up. He assured me he was alright and wanted to go to the restroom. He was not in any way intoxicated. He walked off to use the restroom and after a minute I checked on him and found him lying on his back on the floor. He managed to prop himself up on one elbow and he looked up at me and tried to say something, but he couldn't talk.

I quickly mixed up a 15-drop dose of MMS1, (I try to always carry small bottles with me) and handed it to him. He immediately drank it down. Within five minutes he said, "Boy, that was crazy." Then he sat up. He said before he took the dose everything was going black on him. In 10 minutes he was feeling OK and I was able to help him to his feet. We returned to the table where he asked for a new plate of food and he was fine.

This serves as a wonderful example of how MMS1 can cancel out some poisons right on the spot.

The first step of the Food Poisoning Protocol is a nice big dose of MMS1, along the same lines as for the Malaria Protocol. With poisoning you want to hit it hard with the first dose. But don't expect it to always clear up immediately; you may have to persist a bit. We have helped many cases of food poisoning. It does not always clear up as fast as it did with my friend, but MMS1 has often proven to be successful with cases such as this. You should always carry two small bottles (MMS and activator) with you at all times. Be ready—if you suspect food poisoning or any other kind of poisoning, get some MMS1 into the body as fast as possible.

Instructions for Food Poisoning Protocol

When a person suspects poisoning:

Step 1

❑ Take a 15-drop dose of MMS1 (activated MMS). See page 32 for how to prepare an MMS1 dose.

Step 2

❑ Wait 15 minutes after the first 15-drop dose, and then take a 6-drop dose of MMS1.

Step 3

❑ Wait another 15 minutes and take another 6-drop dose, this would be the third dose. (This means in a 30 minute period, from the starting point, one would have taken 3 doses of MMS. The first and starting dose—15 activated drops. The 2nd and 3rd doses—6 activated drops of MMS.)

Note: *If the person is provoked to vomit during this time—welcome it, do not fight it, for this will help expel the poison from the body. Vomiting may or may not occur if the MMS1 neutralizes all of the poison in the body. It may flush it out without the need to vomit.*

Step 4

❑ If vomiting does not occur while taking the first 3 doses, do not worry. But, take at least 2 more doses (4th and 5th doses); these should be MMS1, 3-drop doses, spaced out by 15 minutes.

Step 5

❑ Normally the above amount of MMS1 will handle the job, but if you are still very sick from poisoning, you may need to take more MMS1 and make yourself vomit. There is nothing wrong with making yourself vomit if you need to do so. In the case of poisoning, vomiting may be necessary in some instances, so don't hesitate if it is needed—it is best to flush the poison out.

❑ You may have to use the old trick of putting your finger down your throat to induce the vomiting. This is not nearly as aggressive as going to an emergency clinic and having your stomach pumped. You can calculate the need to vomit by how sick you still are. If you are still sick you may need to vomit and/or take more MMS1, as there is no down side to taking more MMS1, other than having some nausea and then possibly vomiting, diarrhea, or a headache.

Note: *With poisoning, although unpleasant, vomiting and diarrhea are both efficient ways to rid the body of the toxins.*

Step 6

❑ If after doing all of the above you are still very sick you may need to have your stomach pumped. In that case, don't hesitate; go to a clinic. However, normally under most poisoning conditions, if you have taken the above protocol, you will be OK by this time.

Concussion Protocol

Many people have used DMSO to overcome a concussion. Some managers of sports arenas keep DMSO on hand at all times. The book *DMSO in Trauma and Disease* by the world renowned DMSO research doctor, Dr. Stanley W. Jacob, recommends DMSO in all cases of concussion. Other health practitioners and sports managers also recommend DMSO for the treatment of a concussion.

A concussion is generally considered to be a mild traumatic brain injury, though concussions occur in varying degrees of seriousness. Some symptoms of concussion are:

• Fatigue
• Headaches
• Sleep Disturbances
• Dizziness and Imbalance
• Vision Problems/Extra Sensitivity to Light

- Hearing and Noise Problems
- Muscular and Motor Problems
- Sensory and Metabolic Disturbances
- Chronic Pain Problems
- Sexual Dysfunction
- Seizures

For a number of years now, I have incorporated DMSO along with MMS1 in several of our protocols, as these two complement one another. In the case of a concussion, I suggest doing the following emergency Stroke Protocol.

Stroke Protocol

About 700,000 strokes happen in the United States each year, and of that number approximately 150,000 deaths occur. So strokes are nothing to be ignored. When a stroke is coming on, follow the protocol below. Using DMSO and MMS1 can stop it in its tracks. Both DMSO and MMS1 will dissolve blood clots throughout the body, including in the brain. DMSO has been used in the USA since 1955 and many people have testified about how it has helped overcome strokes. Likewise, DMSO and MMS1 have been used together for an increased benefit by thousands.

Note: *I have been using MMS for 22 years. By the beginning of 2012, I had personally helped over 50,000 people around the world using MMS, (and scores more since that time, but I've lost count). I have only helped one person who was experiencing a stroke, and that was successful. The advice that I give here is what I would do myself if I was having a stroke and a hospital was not available to me. If a hospital was available I would still do this: I would begin the protocol while still at home and I would continue to do it on the way to the hospital, however long it took. When I returned from the hospital, I would continue with* *the protocol. In my opinion, using DMSO and MMS1 might mean the difference between life and death, or the difference between having long term side effects or not. It is nevertheless completely your responsibility to do or not do this protocol.*

Signs of a stroke are:

- **Face Drooping**–Does one side of the face droop or is it numb? Ask the person to smile. Is the person's smile uneven?

- **Arm Weakness**–Is one arm weak or numb? Ask the person to raise both arms. Does one arm drift downward?

- **Speech Difficulty**–Is speech slurred? Is the person unable to speak or hard to understand? Ask the person to repeat a simple sentence, like "The grass is green." Is the sentence repeated correctly?

If someone shows any of these symptoms, even if the symptoms go away, it is time to start the protocol below, or get the person to the hospital immediately if that is their choice. Check the time so you'll know when the first symptoms appeared. In the case of seeking medical assistance, you can still begin with the first doses of DMSO, followed by MMS1 as per the following instructions. Getting DMSO and MMS1 into the body right away may save a life. And if you do this, the person might be OK by the time you are able to get to the hospital. If the decision is made to go to the hospital, it's best to always call an ambulance or get someone else to drive. A person should never attempt to drive himself to a hospital if experiencing a stroke.

Instructions for Overcoming a Stroke with MMS1 and DMSO

Blood clots can cause strokes. DMSO is able to **dissolve blood clots.** MMS1 also works to dissolve clots. Using DMSO in conjunction with MMS1 can be very effective in both overcoming a stroke, as well as repairing damage from a stroke. When a blood clot prevents blood flow to any given area of the brain, a stroke can occur and cause that particular area of the brain to shut down. However, if the blood clot can be dissolved by using DMSO and MMS1, oxygen will once more be able to flow to that area of the brain so that area of the brain can begin to function properly.

Although the instructions below explain what to do at the onset of a stroke, it is important to know that even though a person has already suffered a stroke, and it is a few hours to a day or two later, one can still begin and follow through with these instructions starting at day one (see chart on Dosage Guide for Stroke Protocol Day 1). There is still hope that damage can be avoided or reversed. It has been reported that even though many months or a couple of years have passed after a stroke, if one will go on a regular regimen of taking DMSO along with MMS1, it may reverse part or all of the damage.

The taste of DMSO is far from enjoyable. However, the benefit of using it far outweighs the bad taste. The pharmaceutical grade DMSO has been described as having almost no smell or bad taste. It can be found on the internet and in some pharmacies. The cost is substantially higher.

Day 1—at the Onset of a Stroke

The instructions below are very detailed. We have included a Dosage Guide Chart at the end of this section to help facilitate one following this protocol. However, please do not cut corners and proceed straight to the chart; thoroughly read all of the instructions below to gain a good understanding of the procedure.

First Hour

❑ **At the onset of a stroke**, first off, mix 2 full tablespoons (30 ml) of DMSO diluted in 1/2 cup (4 ounces/120 ml) of water. Drink it down immediately. This is the **starting point** of the Stroke Protocol.

❑ **Also at the onset of a stroke,** begin Protocol 6 and 6. This is two 6-drop doses of activated MMS (MMS1), taken one hour apart. (See page 169 for full details of Protocol 6 and 6.) MMS1 and DMSO work in conjunction with one another, therefore the first 6-drop dose of MMS1 for a stroke, should be taken in less than two minutes after the first dose of DMSO. The MMS1 must be mixed up in a second 1/2 cup (4 ounces/120 ml) of water. (It should be taken right after the DMSO dose, but do not mix in with the DMSO.) If at any time you miss the two-minute limit, always go ahead and take the dose even if three, five, ten minutes or more have passed. Try not to miss the two-minute limit.

❑ **Fifteen minutes after the starting point** of this protocol, one should take a second dose of 2 tablespoons (30 ml) of DMSO in 1/2 cup (4 ounces/120 ml) of water. No MMS1 is taken at this time.

❑ **Thirty minutes after the starting point**, a third 2 tablespoon (30 ml) dose of DMSO in 1/2 cup (4 ounces/120 ml) of water should be taken. No MMS1 is taken at this time.

❑ **Forty-five minutes after the starting point**, a fourth 2 tablespoon (30 ml) dose of DMSO in 1/2 cup

(4 ounces/120 ml) should be taken. No MMS1 is taken at this time.

Second Hour

❑ **One hour after starting** this stroke protocol, (which is the beginning of the second hour), continue to take DMSO every 15 minutes, reduce the dosage to 1 tablespoon (15 ml) of DMSO in 1/4 cup (2 ounces/60 ml) of water.

❑ **Also one hour after starting** this stroke protocol, within two minutes time of taking the DMSO dose, take another 6-drop dose of MMS1. This is the second 6-drop dose, taken one hour after the first 6-drop dose. Do not take more than two 6-drop doses of MMS1, one hour a part.

Third Hour

❑ **Two hours after the starting point**, (which will be the beginning of the third hour), take another DMSO dose. Continue taking 1 tablespoon (15 ml) of DMSO in 1/4 cup (2 ounces/60 ml) of water every 15 minutes the third hour.

❑ **Also two hours after the starting point,** at the beginning of the third hour, begin taking Protocol 1000. This is a 3-drop dose of MMS1 every hour for eight hours a day. This 3-drop dose of MMS1, should be taken within two minutes of the first DMSO dose at the beginning of the third hour.

❑ Generally I suggest gradually working up to the 3-drop dose when beginning Protocol 1000. Going right to 3 drops an hour for the Stroke Protocol, is an exception to the rule. If however, one experiences a Herxheimer reaction and feels nauseated, has diarrhea or vomits, cut the MMS1 dose in half. If necessary, keep reducing it by one half until these symptoms subside. When the symptoms pass, gradually work back up to a 3-drop dose every hour, or to as high a dose that is comfortable to you without causing a Herxheimer reaction. But do not surpass more than 3 drops an hour while on Protocol 1000.

Notes

➤ *Remember, if a person is led to lower their dose of MMS1, they should lower it, but do not quit taking it altogether.*

➤ *Up until this point, the person on this protocol will have completed three hours in total of taking DMSO every 15 minutes.*

➤ *Please take note that when you **lower the amount of DMSO in your dose, it is important to also lower the amount of water you mix with it.***

Fourth through Eighth Hour

❑ **After the first three hours** of taking DMSO every 15 minutes in the different dosages described above, continue taking DMSO for the remaining part of the first day, but reduce the frequency of your doses. One time every hour take 1 tablespoon (15 ml) of DMSO in 1/4 cup (2 ounces/60 ml) of water. The person should already have started taking Protocol 1000, which is an hourly 3-drop dose of MMS1. The hourly DMSO dose and the hourly MMS1 dose should always be taken within two minutes (maximum) apart.

Notes

➤ ***Do not mix the MMS1 dose in with the DMSO mixture.*** *Do not confuse this with other protocols where it does call for adding DMSO drops into the MMS1 dose. In this case, the dose of DMSO is much higher than in other protocols, therefore it is recommended to not mix DMSO in the same dose with MMS1.* **Take the MMS1 dose in less than two minutes time** *after the DMSO dose, but separately, not in the same cup of water.*

➤ *We have mentioned here what to do on "day one" at the onset of a stroke. However, a stroke can strike at any time, and should one feel a stroke coming on in the evening, for example, it would be wise to follow the dosing mentioned above, into the night. In other words, stay up or set an alarm if you have to, in order to take your doses, as strokes can afflict people in their sleep.*

Day 2 through 7

❑ The second day after a stroke, and after one has followed the procedure for day one above, continue taking MMS1, as per Protocol 1000. This is taking a 3-drop dose of MMS1 every hour for eight consecutive hours. I recommend completing the suggested three full weeks of doing Protocol 1000, even if one starts to feel much better, as a precautionary measure.

❑ The second day after a stroke, one can reduce the DMSO intake to 1 tablespoon (15 ml) in the morning and 1 tablespoon (15 ml) in the evening. This amount of DMSO should be taken in 1/4 cup (2 ounces/60 ml) of water. These DMSO dosages should be taken in coordination with the MMS1 dosage. One should be on Protocol 1000, so I suggest they take the DMSO dose within two minutes of the first MMS1 dose of the day, and the last MMS1 dose of the day.

Day 8 through 21

❑ Continue Protocol 1000, until you complete the 21-day period.

❑ Drop your intake of DMSO to taking 1 tablespoon (15 ml) of DMSO only 1 time a day (within two minutes of one of your MMS1 doses), for the remaining 21 days.

❑ If you feel you are not making progress in your recovery, I recommend going back to day one of the Stroke Protocol and starting the whole process over again, as outlined above. In other words, start from the beginning and again continue through until you have completed the 21 days.

Notes

➤ *If one has had a stroke and has recovered fully, I nevertheless recommend a daily maintenance dose of MMS1 (6-drop dose) and 1 tablespoon (15 ml) of DMSO in 1/4 cup (2 ounces/60ml) of water. If at any time the symptoms of a stroke come on again, the complete procedure outlined above should be followed.*

➤ *Take a look at your diet and exercise habits to see if there is room for improvement.*

➤ *Unfortunately, there is no complete guarantee of recovery from a stroke. However many people have recovered from strokes using DMSO, and MMS1 has also been a help in this area.*

Following are two charts to guide you through this protocol. It is important that you start hour 00:00 immediately when needed and continue with the 15 minute intervals from your starting point (e.g. if a stroke comes on at 12:20 pm start taking DMSO and MMS1 immediately, then 15 minutes later would be 12:35 pm and so on).

Dosage Guide for Stroke Protocol Day 1

Start hour 00:00 immediately whenever it is needed, regardless of the actual time. Do not Wait.

Step	Hour	Hour/Min.	MMS1	DMSO/Water
1	Start Hour 1	00:00	6 Drops	2 Tbsp (30 ml) 4 oz (120 ml)
2		00:15	0	2 Tbsp (30 ml) 4 oz (120 ml)
3		00:30	0	2 Tbsp (30 ml) 4 oz (120 ml)
4		00:45	0	2 Tbsp (30 ml) 4 oz (120 ml)
5	Hour 2	01:00	6 Drops	1 Tbsp (15 ml) 2 oz (60 ml)
6		01:15	0	1 Tbsp (15 ml) 2 oz (60 ml)
7		01:30	0	1 Tbsp (15 ml) 2 oz (60 ml)
8		01:45	0	1 Tbsp (15 ml) 2 oz (60 ml)
9	Hour 3	02:00	3 Drops	1 Tbsp (15 ml) 2 oz (60 ml)
10		02:15	0	1 Tbsp (15 ml) 2 oz (60 ml)
11		02:30	0	1 Tbsp (15 ml) 2 oz (60 ml)
12		02:45	0	1 Tbsp (15 ml) 2 oz (60 ml)
13	Hour 4	03:00	3 Drops	1 Tbsp (15 ml) 2 oz (60 ml)
14	Hour 5	04:00	3 Drops	1 Tbsp (15 ml) 2 oz (60 ml)
15	Hour 6	05:00	3 Drops	1 Tbsp (15 ml) 2 oz (60 ml)
16	Hour 7	06:00	3 Drops	1 Tbsp (15 ml) 2 oz (60 ml)
17	Hour 8	07:00	3 Drops	1 Tbsp (15 ml) 2 oz (60 ml)

Dosage Guide for Stroke Protocol Day 2 – 7				
Step	Hour	Hour/ Min.	MMS1	DMSO/ Water
1	Start Hour 1	00:00	3 Drops	1 Tbsp (15 ml) 2 oz (60 ml)
2	Hour 2	01:00	3 Drops	0
3	Hour 3	02:00	3 Drops	0
4	Hour 4	03:00	3 Drops	0
5	Hour 5	04:00	3 Drops	0
6	Hour 6	05:00	3 Drops	0
7	Hour 7	06:00	3 Drops	0
8	Hour 8	07:00	3 Drops	1 Tbsp (15 ml) 2 oz (60 ml)

Day 8 – 21

- Continue with Protocol 1000, until you complete the 21-day period.
- Drop your dose of DMSO from 2 tablespoons (30 ml) to taking 1 tablespoon (15 ml) of DMSO daily, for the remaining 21 days.
- If not making progress, go back to Day 1. Start the whole process over again.
- Refer to complete protocol on page 227 for details.

Heart Attack Protocol

About 600,000 heart attack deaths happen in the US each year. When a heart attack is coming on, following the combined DMSO/MMS1 protocol below, can stop it in its tracks. DMSO has been used in the US since 1955 and there are many testimonies about how it has helped overcome heart attacks. In addition, MMS1 has been used extensively since the year 2000, and DMSO and MMS1 have both been used together for an increased benefit by thousands.

Note: *I have been using MMS for 22 years. By the begin-ning of 2012, I had personally helped over 50,000 people around the world using MMS, (and scores more since that time, but I've lost count). I have only helped three people who were experiencing a heart attack, each case was successful. The advice that I give here is what I would do myself if I was having a heart attack and a hospital was not available to me. If a hospital was available, I would still do this: I would begin the protocol while still at home and I would continue to do it on the way to the hospital, however long it took. When I returned from the hospital, I would continue with the protocol. In my opinion, using DMSO and MMS1 might mean the difference between life and death, or the difference between having long term side effects or not. It is nevertheless completely your responsibility to do or not do this protocol.*

Signs of a heart attack are pain in the chest, arms, (especially the left), back, neck, jaw, and upper stomach; and shortness of breath, nausea, lightheadedness, and cold sweats.

If one suspects a heart attack coming on, it's time to start on the protocols, or get the person to the hospital imme-diately if that is their choice. Check the time so you'll know when the first symptoms appeared. In the case of seeking medical assistance, you can still begin with the first doses of DMSO, followed by MMS1 as per the instructions below. Getting DMSO and MMS1 into the body right away may save a life. And if you do this, the person might be OK by the time you are able to get to the hospital. If the decision is made to go to the hospital, it's best to always call an ambulance or get someone else to drive. A person should never attempt to drive oneself to a hospital if experiencing a heart attack.

Instructions for Overcoming a Heart Attack with MMS1 and DMSO

Although the instructions below explain what to do at the onset of a heart attack, it is important to know that even though a person has already suffered a heart attack, and it is a few hours to a day or two later, one can still begin and follow through with these instructions starting at day one (see chart on Dosage Guide for Heart Attack Protocol Day 1, page 244). There is still hope that damage can be avoided or reversed. If one will go on a regular regimen of taking DMSO along with MMS1, it may reverse part or all of the damage.

The taste of DMSO is far from enjoyable. However, the benefit of using it far outweighs the bad taste. The pharmaceutical grade DMSO has been described as having **almost** no smell or bad taste. It can be found on the internet and in some pharmacies. The cost is substantially higher.

Day 1—at the Onset of a Heart Attack

The instructions below are very detailed. We have included a Dosage Guide Chart at the end of this section to help facilitate one following this protocol. However, please do not cut corners and proceed straight to the chart, thoroughly read all of the instructions below to gain a good understanding of the procedure.

First Hour

❑ **At the onset of a heart attack**, first off, mix 2 full tablespoons (30 ml) of DMSO diluted in 1/2 cup (4 ounces/120 ml) of water. Drink it down immediately. This is the **starting point** of the Heart Attack Protocol.

❑ **Also at the onset of a heart attack,** begin Protocol 6 and 6. This is two 6-drop doses of activated MMS (MMS1), taken one hour apart. (See page 169 for full details of Protocol 6 and 6.) MMS1 and DMSO work in conjunction with one another, therefore the first 6-drop dose of MMS1 for a heart attack, should be taken in less than two minutes after the first dose of DMSO. The MMS1 must be mixed up in a second 1/2 cup (4 ounces/120 ml) of water. (It should be taken right after the DMSO dose, but do not mix in with the DMSO.) If at any time you miss the two-minute limit, always go ahead and take the dose even if three, five, ten minutes or more have passed. Try not to miss the two-minute limit.

❑ **Fifteen minutes after the starting point** of this protocol, one should take a second dose of 2 tablespoons (30 ml) of DMSO in 1/2 cup (4 ounces/120 ml) of water. No MMS1 is taken at this time.

❑ **Thirty minutes after the starting point**, a third 2 tablespoon (30 ml) dose of DMSO in 1/2 cup (4 ounces/120 ml) of water should be taken. No MMS1 is taken at this time.

❑ **Forty-five minutes after the starting point**, a fourth 2 tablespoon (30 ml) dose of DMSO in 1/2 cup (4 ounces/120 ml) should be taken. No MMS1 is taken at this time.

Second Hour

❑ **One hour after starting** this heart attack protocol, (which is the beginning of the second hour), continue to take DMSO every 15 minutes, but reduce the dosage to 1 tablespoon (15 ml) of DMSO in 1/4 cup (2 ounces/60 ml) of water.

❏ **Also one hour after starting** this heart attack protocol, within two minutes time of taking the DMSO dose, take another 6-drop dose of MMS1. This is the second 6-drop dose, taken one hour after the first 6-drop dose. Do not take more than two 6-drop doses of MMS1, one hour a part.

Third Hour

❏ **Two hours after the starting point**, (which will be the beginning of the third hour), take another DMSO dose. Continue taking 1 tablespoon (15 ml) of DMSO in 1/4 cup (2 ounces/60 ml) of water every 15 minutes the third hour.

❏ **Also two hours after the starting point,** at the beginning of the third hour, begin taking Protocol 1000. This is a 3-drop dose of MMS1 every hour for eight hours a day. This 3-drop dose of MMS1, should be taken within two minutes of the first DMSO dose at the beginning of the third hour.

❏ Generally I suggest gradually working up to the 3-drop dose when beginning Protocol 1000. Going right to 3 drops an hour for the Heart Protocol, is an exception to the rule. If however, one experiences a Herxheimer reaction and feels nauseated, has diarrhea or vomits, cut the MMS1 dose in half. If necessary, keep reducing it by one half until these symptoms subside. When the symptoms pass, gradually work back up to a 3-drop dose every hour, or to as high a dose that is comfortable to you without causing a Herxheimer reaction. But do not surpass more than 3 drops an hour while on Protocol 1000.

Notes

➤   *Remember, if a person is led to lower the dose of MMS1, they should lower it, but do not quit taking it altogether.*

➤   *Up until this point, the person on this protocol will have completed three hours in total of taking DMSO every 15 minutes.*

➤   *Please take note that **when you lower the amount of DMSO in your dose, it is important to also lower the amount of water you mix with it.***

Fourth through Eighth Hour

❑   **After the first three hours** of taking DMSO every 15 minutes in the different dosages described above, continue taking DMSO for the remaining part of the first day, but reduce the frequency of your doses. One time every hour take 1 tablespoon (15 ml) of DMSO in 1/4 cup (2 ounces/60 ml) of water. The person should already have started taking Protocol 1000, which is an hourly 3-drop dose of MMS1. The hourly DMSO dose and the hourly MMS1 dose should always be taken within two minutes (maximum) apart.

Notes

➤   ***Do not mix the MMS1 dose in with the DMSO mixture.*** *Do not confuse this with other protocols where it does call for adding DMSO drops into the MMS1 dose. In this case, the dose of DMSO is much higher than in other protocols, therefore it is recommended to not mix DMSO in the same dose with MMS1. **Take the MMS1 dose in less than two minutes time** after the DMSO dose, but separately, not in the same cup of water.*

> ➤ *We have mentioned here what to do on "day one" at the onset of a heart attack. However, a heart attack can strike at any time, and should one feel a heart attack coming on in the evening, for example, it would be wise to follow the dosing mentioned above, into the night. In other words, stay up or set an alarm if you have to, in order to take your doses, as a heart attack can afflict people in their sleep.*

Day 2 through 7

❑ The second day after a heart attack, and after one has followed the procedure for day one above, continue taking MMS1, as per Protocol 1000. This is taking a 3-drop dose of MMS1 every hour for eight consecutive hours. I recommend completing the suggested three full weeks of doing Protocol 1000, even if one starts to feel much better, as a precautionary measure.

❑ The second day after a heart attack, one can reduce the DMSO intake to 1 tablespoon (15 ml) in the morning and 1 tablespoon (15 ml) in the evening. This amount of DMSO should be taken in 1/4 cup (2 ounces/60 ml) of water. These DMSO dosages should be taken in coordination with the MMS1 dosage. One should be on Protocol 1000, so I suggest they take the DMSO dose within two minutes of the first MMS1 dose of the day, and the last MMS1 dose of the day.

Day 8 through 21

❑ Continue Protocol 1000, until you complete the 21-day period.

❑ Drop your intake of DMSO to taking 1 tablespoon (15 ml) of DMSO only 1 time a day (within two minutes of one of your MMS1 doses), for the remaining 21 days.

❑ If you feel you are not making progress in your recovery, I recommend going back to day one of the Heart Attack Protocol and starting the whole process over again, as outlined above. In other words, start from the beginning and again continue through until you have completed the 21 days.

Notes

➤ *If one has had a heart attack and has recovered fully, I nevertheless recommend a daily maintenance dose of MMS1 (6-drop dose) and 1 tablespoon (15 ml) of DMSO in 1/4 cup (2 ounces/60ml) of water. If at any time the symptoms of a heart attack come on again, the complete procedure outlined above should be followed.*

➤ *Take a look at your diet and exercise habits to see if there is room for improvement.*

➤ *Unfortunately, there is no guarantee of recovery from a heart attack, but thousands of people have recovered from heart attacks using DMSO, and MMS1 has also been a help in this area.*

Following are two charts to guide you through this protocol. It is important that you start hour 00:00 immediately when needed and continue with the 15 minute intervals from your starting point (e.g. if a heart attack comes on at 12:20 pm start taking DMSO and MMS1 immediately, then 15 minutes later would be 12:35 pm and so on).

Dosage Guide for Heart Attack Protocol Day 1

Start hour 00:00 immediately whenever it is needed, regardless of the actual time. Do not Wait.

Step	Hour	Hour/ Min.	MMS1	DMSO/ Water
1	Start Hour 1	00:00	6 Drops	2 Tbsp (30 ml) 4 oz (120 ml)
2		00:15	0	2 Tbsp (30 ml) 4 oz (120 ml)
3		00:30	0	2 Tbsp (30 ml) 4 oz (120 ml)
4		00:45	0	2 Tbsp (30 ml) 4 oz (120 ml)
5	Hour 2	01:00	6 Drops	1 Tbsp (15 ml) 2 oz (60 ml)
6		01:15	0	1 Tbsp (15 ml) 2 oz (60 ml)
7		01:30	0	1 Tbsp (15 ml) 2 oz (60 ml)
8		01:45	0	1 Tbsp (15 ml) 2 oz (60 ml)
9	Hour 3	02:00	3 Drops	1 Tbsp (15 ml) 2 oz (60 ml)
10		02:15	0	1 Tbsp (15 ml) 2 oz (60 ml)
11		02:30	0	1 Tbsp (15 ml) 2 oz (60 ml)
12		02:45	0	1 Tbsp (15 ml) 2 oz (60 ml)
13	Hour 4	03:00	3 Drops	1 Tbsp (15 ml) 2 oz (60 ml)
14	Hour 5	04:00	3 Drops	1 Tbsp (15 ml) 2 oz (60 ml)
15	Hour 6	05:00	3 Drops	1 Tbsp (15 ml) 2 oz (60 ml)
16	Hour 7	06:00	3 Drops	1 Tbsp (15 ml) 2 oz (60 ml)
17	Hour 8	07:00	3 Drops	1 Tbsp (15 ml) 2 oz (60 ml)

Dosage Guide for Heart Attack Protocol Day 2 – 7				
Step	Hour	Hour/ Min.	MMS1	DMSO/ Water
1	Start Hour 1	00:00	3 Drops	1 Tbsp (15 ml) 2 oz (60 ml)
2	Hour 2	01:00	3 Drops	0
3	Hour 3	02:00	3 Drops	0
4	Hour 4	03:00	3 Drops	0
5	Hour 5	04:00	3 Drops	0
6	Hour 6	05:00	3 Drops	0
7	Hour 7	06:00	3 Drops	0
8	Hour 8	07:00	3 Drops	1 Tbsp (15 ml) 2 oz (60 ml)

Day 8 – 21

- Continue with Protocol 1000, until you complete the 21-day period.
- Drop your dose of DMSO from 2 tablespoons (30 ml) to taking 1 tablespoon (15 ml) of DMSO daily, for the remaining 21 days.
- If not making progress, go back to Day 1. Start the whole process over again.
- Refer to complete protocol on page 236 for details.

Burn Protocol

Burns cause acid to be generated in the skin and tissues which were burned. Unactivated MMS (22.4% solution of sodium chlorite in water) is highly alkaline and alkaline water cancels acid, thus when one gently rubs **unactivated** MMS onto the burn most of the acid will be neutralized which will eliminate much of the pain. The acid in the burn may activate some of the sodium chlorite in the MMS, thus oxidizing some of the burn poisons and also reducing the pain. Normally the pain is gone instantly or in a few minutes when using *unactivated* MMS, but sometimes on very bad burns it can take longer. Healing time for burns when *unactivated* MMS is used can be up to 4 times faster than normal. The following protocol can be used for first, second and third degree burns.

Please note this protocol is an **exception** to the overall rule of activating MMS with a food grade acid. I recommend using unactivated MMS in a very small amount, directly on a mosquito bite and some other insect bites (see pages 196, 206-208). I likewise recommend using unactivated MMS for burns, (the amount depends on the size of the burn). If using unactivated MMS for a burn, please follow the explicit instructions below. In general, for all other protocols in this book, we recommend activating MMS with a food grade acid, then adding the indicated amount of water before use.

Instructions for Burns—Using Unactivated MMS

Step 1

❑ In case of a burn anywhere on the body, immediately, or as soon as possible, put plenty of unactivated MMS on the burned area. (If the burn is on the face, take care to avoid the eyes.) Don't be concerned about getting a little unactivated MMS on unburned skin. (See below: You will be washing it off in five minutes.)

❑ With your fingertips gently rub (barely touching the burn but enough to make sure of contact) the MMS directly into the burn. The pain will begin to diminish immediately.

Step 2

❑ **Do not allow unactivated MMS to remain on your skin for more than five minutes!** It must be rinsed off with clean, cool or cold water. If you forget and allow the MMS to remain on the burn it will aggravate the burn and the healing will take longer than usual.

Step 3

❑ Depending upon the severity of the burn, the pain normally will stop within five minutes. If the pain is not completely gone at the end of five minutes, you can apply a second amount of unactivated MMS, but only after rinsing off the first application. Follow the exact procedure as outlined in Steps 1 and 2 above.

Notes

➤ *In the case of severe burns, if you have applied 2 applications of unactivated MMS and the pain continues, you can then apply unactivated MMS every one-half hour for up to two hours. (But remember, each application must be rinsed off after five minutes.)*

➤ *If the pain still continues after this two hour period, you can apply unactivated MMS two more times, but this time, one hour apart. Each of these applications should be according to Steps 1 and 2 above.*

➤ *In general, the pain will be gone within four hours, but if not, you can continue the process outlined in Steps 1 and 2 every four hours.*

➤ *After the pain subsides, if you have access to fresh Aloe vera, this can help aid healing a burn. Slice open (length-wise) one leaf of the fresh plant and apply the fresh gel to the burn area. This can be repeated as often as necessary.*

Caution! Remember, **never leave unactivated MMS on your skin for longer than five minutes,** always rinse it off with cool water.

Instructions for Sunburns—Using Unactivated MMS

Step 1

❏ In case of sunburn, either severe or a very light case, it is best to spray unactivated MMS directly on the burned area.

❏ After spraying, very gently rub the unactivated MMS over the burned skin.

Step 2

❏ Be sure to rinse the MMS off with clean cool or cold water in five minutes or less. Do not allow it to remain on the skin more than five minutes or it will cause your skin to peel.

Step 3

❏ With sunburn, some pain may start up again in several hours, in this case apply unactivated MMS again, but for no longer than five minutes, then rinse off with clean, cool or cold water.

Notes

➤ *Sunburn is different than other burns as it is mostly more on the surface of the skin, therefore it is treated differently.* **Do not apply unactivated MMS more than 5 times in total to sunburn,** *and* **not more than one time per hour.** *Never let it remain on your skin longer than five minutes.*

➤ *In general, sunburn clears up in one hour, up to one day.*

One Week to Live Protocol

If the doctor says you only have one or two weeks left to live, I would say it's worth giving MMS a try. Why not? Medical science has not worked and there is nothing left to lose. I have received emails from many people stating that they have revived from near death, when according to doctors they had only a week or two left. There are no guarantees in life. But never give up on yourself or someone else. Even if a person only has one hour left, get some MMS into the body.

In the event a person has one to two weeks to live, I would suggest to fast-track the HRP as follows:

The Starting Procedure

Begin the Starting Procedure, but in this case, remove all the stops. Ultra fast-track the Starting Procedure—do it in one day, go through each step.

❑ Take a 1/4-drop dose for two hours.

❑ Increase to a 1/2-drop dose for the next two hours.

❑ Increase to a 3/4-drop dose for the next two hours.

❑ Lastly, increase to a 1-drop dose for another two hours.

Notes

➤ *This is eight hours in total of taking MMS1, increasing the intake from 1/4 drop to 1 drop over that period of time.*

➤ *At any time during this process if you experience an additional feeling of sickness, cut back the dose by 1/2 the amount of your last dose. For example if a 1/2-drop dose makes you feel sick, cut back again to 1/4 of a drop. Begin increasing the drops again when you feel your body is able to tolerate more. If this should be the case, it may take longer than one day to get through the Starting Procedure. Be attentive to how the body is reacting and adjust the dose accordingly.*

Protocol 1000, 1000 Plus and 2000

After you have fast-tracked the Starting Procedure, the idea is to move on to Protocol 1000 and proceed to Protocol 1000 Plus and to Protocol 2000 as quickly as you can, but without allowing yourself to feel worse than your illness is already making you feel.

❑ After completing the fast-track Starting Procedure outlined above, go on to Protocol 1000. Start out with a 1-drop dose the first hour and increase the drops with each dose, according to what your body can tolerate, until you reach 3 drops per dose.

❑ When you reach a 3-drop dose, if everything is going well and you are not experiencing any additional sickness, after three to four 3-drop doses of MMS1, you can begin to add DMSO to your doses (as per Protocol 1000 Plus instructions).

❑ After taking 2 to 3 doses of MMS1 with DMSO added, proceed on to Protocol 2000 as quickly as your body can handle it. This means keep increasing the amount of MMS1 drops and DMSO with each hourly dose according to what your body can tolerate. (The ratio of DMSO to MMS1 is 3 drops of DMSO to every 1 drop of MMS1.) If you do not have DMSO do not let that stop you, just continue to increase the MMS1 drops every hour.

❏ After two days of increasing MMS1 and DMSO drops, again, if all is going well, add in MMS2 as per instructions in Protocol 2000.

❏ At any time during this process if you experience additional sickness, cut back the dose by 1/2 the amount of your last dose. Begin increasing the drops again when you feel your body is able to tolerate more. You want to find the right amount of drops that you can tolerate without feeling worse than you already feel.

Notes

➤ *Remember the Golden Rules of MMS (see pages 83-84), especially the one that says that any time you see improvement do not change anything; continue with what you are doing. Although this protocol is suggesting to fast-track, nevertheless, if you are getting better, stick with what you are doing. As long as you are improving, stay at that dosage of MMS1, DSMO and MMS2, whatever point you are at—whatever dosage brings improvement, keep doing it. When you reach a point where you do not see any improvement for a one or two day period, increase your intake, moving to the next level.*

➤ *Do not take vitamins or supplements during this time. Wait until the disease pathogens are eradicated, then you can work on building up your nutrition.*

Protocol 3000

❏ You can add Protocol 3000 as soon as possible while taking the oral doses mentioned above, unless you are already improving, in which case it is not necessary to go to Protocol 3000.

❑ But when you do not see any improvement for a one to two day period, add Protocol 3000 to what you are already doing.

Supporting Protocols

❑ Add on any of the Supporting Protocols one at a time, especially if they are in line with helping your particular illness. For example, if the problem is colon cancer, add on enemas. If the problem is ovarian cancer, add on douches. If the problem is skin cancer, use the spray bottle and so on.

❑ Continue with Supporting Protocols if they seem to be helping, but back off any time they do not seem to be helping.

Unconscious or Cannot Swallow

Do not give MMS to someone who is unconscious or cannot swallow. It is possible to administer MMS through an IV drip. I do not recommend this, or the following tube method, unless a qualified person is overseeing the procedure. For an IV drip use a 250 ml bag of IV saline or glucose solution. Put 20 drops of activated MMS into the solution. Regulate the drip so that it goes into the body over a period of one hour. This can be repeated several times a day, but other applicable supporting and additional protocols should also be used.

If the person has a feeding tube you can give him MMS doses right through the tube. Mix the appropriate dose of MMS1 (according to what protocol the person is on) and pour the dose into the tube. This can be done on an hourly basis. Follow the Starting Procedure as outlined above in this protocol and continue on to the other protocols as instructed.

Depending on the situation, in the case of someone who is unconscious or who cannot swallow here are other ways to get MMS into the body: Protocol 3000 (external application of DMSO and MMS1). The Bag Protocol is another option if they are conscious but have a problem with swallowing. If using the bag, make absolutely sure that the person cannot get a breath of the gas as that could cause harm. Depending on the circumstances one may also be able to do an MMS bath. (A foot bath could also be helpful if the person is unable to get into a bathtub.) If you are the one who is sick, you will need someone to help you, preferably someone who is knowledgeable about MMS. But if for some reason that person is not available, hire someone you feel confident can help you and have them read this book.

Brown Recluse: I got bit by a Brown Recluse spider, my leg was getting so bad I couldn't walk. The doctors would not help other than antibiotics and a friend suggested MMS, so I put some on the bite which was rotting from the spiders toxins. The next day all the dead flesh from the spider bite just fell right out of my leg when I rinsed it with water and the wound healed immediately after. Thanks Jim! —A

Scorpion and more: In Indonesia I used MMS very effectively for: Scorpion, hornet, wasp, centipede bites, flu, diarrhea, reef cuts, ear infection and some more. —T. I.

AIDS: A few years ago a mature woman with full blown AIDS was brought to our church for prayer. My pastor asked me to help her. Since she had already declined to take the anti retroviral medication on her own accord, I put her on Protocol 1000. I also gave her my soft-bounce mini trampoline. Since she could not walk on her own, I gave instructions for her relatives to assist her on the trampoline until she could bounce on her own. She also had several healing scriptures which she had to read 8 times daily, just as with the use of MMS and the trampoline.

Two weeks later a woman fitting the description of a gym instructor strode into our prayer meeting. It took some convincing to confirm that this was the same shadow of a woman with full blown AIDS! We were dumbfounded: It's TRUE! MMS is the real deal! I knew MMS works—but not this fast—and so thorough. That very day she had jumped on the trampoline for 1 1/2 hrs! She explained that while the 1st week was exceptionally challenging, she persevered and felt enormously better at the beginning of the 2nd week...and she was only at 2 drops per hour! MMS is a stand-alone powerhouse, and makes other protocols work incredibly better! —Stephen, Trinidad/Tobago

Multiple Uses: We have used MMS here in Australia for few years now on many health problems—flu, spider bites, teeth infection, cuts, food poisoning, water cleansing on trips to the bush—also given to friends for other ills. Over the years none of us have any side effects at all. It's very safe if you follow G2 protocol. —JPR

Chapter 13

Adjusting Protocol Dosages for Children

A Word to Parents

In this book we assume that every parent is totally responsible for their children's health. Ideally, if you are going to give MMS to a child, you should have enough experience with it to have used it yourself first. Read this book in its entirety and check out some of the links in the back of the book for more information and testimonies.

However, if there is an emergency concerning your child, you may just have to trust the information in these pages and follow these directions, if you so choose, even if you haven't used MMS yourself.

We have written this book taking extreme care to make it understandable for you, but we expect each person to take full responsibility for their use of the data. We have done our very best to bring you the latest available information on MMS. The protocols in this book have been fine-tuned as a result of receiving feedback from thousands of worldwide MMS users.

When giving MMS protocols to children, the same principles apply to them as for adults. For example, if a protocol calls for hourly doses for an adult, it would also call for hourly doses for a child. Taking MMS hourly is important.

Also, if the child becomes nauseated or has diarrhea, reduce the dose by 50% (or more if necessary) until the problem subsides and then increase back up to the proper amount indicated for the particular protocol the child is on.

The thing that varies for children is the dosage size—the **number** of drops you give, or the **size** of the capsule. The amount of MMS1 and MMS2 you give a child is determined by the weight of the child. Following are instructions on how to determine the amount of MMS1 and MMS2 for children to take when on various protocols in this book.

Starting Procedure for Children

The Starting Procedure should always be done before a child goes on to Protocol 1000. For further information on the Starting Procedure, including how to measure a fraction of a drop, see pages 80-81, and follow the details given there.

Starting Procedure MMS1 Dosage Guide for Children				
Drops Per Hour	**Day 1**	**Day 2**	**Day 3**	**Day 4**
Babies less than 7 lbs (3.2 kg)	1/8 drop	1/8 drop	1/4 drop	1/2 drop
Children 7-24 lbs (3.2-11 kg)	1/8 drop	1/4 drop	1/4 drop	1/2 drop
Children 25-49 lbs (11-23 kg)	1/4 drop	1/4 drop	1/2 drop	3/4 drop
Children 50-74 lbs (23-34 kg)	1/4 drop	1/2 drop	1/2 drop	3/4 drop
Children 75-100 lbs (34-45 kg)	1/4 drop	1/2 drop	1/2 drop	3/4 drop

Protocol 1000 for Children

Protocol 1000 is taking a dose of MMS1 every hour for eight consecutive hours a day. The maximum adult dose for Protocol 1000 is 3 drops of MMS1 per hour; however, please remember, as per the instructions for this protocol starting on page 86, one must **work up** to the 3-drop dose. This same principle applies to children.

The basic rule of thumb for dosing children with MMS1 is when the child weighs above 25 lbs (11 kg), give 1 drop of MMS1 (activated MMS) for every additional 25 lbs. However, we have provided charts for determining dosing. Please use these charts. And again, remember the golden rule of MMS—whenever a child (or anybody for that matter) becomes nauseated, has diarrhea or experiences discomfort beyond what the sickness is already causing, cut back the dosage by 50%, or more if needed, until the symptoms subside and then work back up to the proper dosing for the weight of the child. Generally this would be in one to three days.

Never go beyond these amounts of drops per hour, as per the child's respective weight, while on Protocol 1000.

Note: *For how to make a 1/4, 1/2, or 3/4 drop dose see the Starting Procedure (pages 80-81). To make a dose that is 1-1/2 drop, make a 2-drop dose of MMS1 in 1/2 cup (4 ounces/120 ml) of water. Pour off 1 ounce of the liquid (or 1/4 of the 1/2 cup) and you will have a dose that equals 1-1/2 drop.*

Protocol 1000 MMS1 Dosage Guide for Children	
Weight	**MMS1 Drops Per Hour**
Babies weighing less than 7 lbs (3.2 kg)	1/2 drop per hour the first day of Protocol 1000, then work up to 3/4 drop per hour for the remaining 21-day period of protocol.
Children 7-24 lbs (3.2-10 kg)	1/2 drop per hour to start and work up to 1 drop per hour for the remaining 21-day period.
Children 25-49 lbs (11-22 kg)	Start with 3/4 drop per hour and work up to 1-1/2 drops per hour for the remaining 21-day period.
Children 50-74 lbs (22-33 kg)	Start at 1 drop per hour and work up to 2 drops per hour for the remaining 21-day period.
Children 75 lbs (34 kg) and over	Start at 1 drop per hour and work up to 3 drops per hour for the remaining 21-day period.

Protocol 1000 Plus for Children

Protocol 1000 Plus for children, is the same ratio as for an adult dose when adding DMSO. That is, for every 1 drop of MMS1 (activated MMS) you give a child, add 3 drops of DMSO. Be sure to diligently read the section for Protocol 1000 Plus, page 87, to be sure you are mixing the dose correctly and adding DMSO at the right time.

Protocol 2000 for Children

Protocol 2000 for a child works the same as for Protocol 2000 for an adult, but again, the amount of MMS1 and MMS2 for a child will be different than that of an adult. Please read the section on Protocol 2000, page 89, as well as the section on MMS2 Details, on page 274.

When on Protocol 2000, give a child as much MMS1 as he/she can tolerate **(but do not exceed the maximum amounts in the chart below)** without adding to the sickness the illness is already causing. This requires very careful observation of the child. Be ready to reduce the dose if there are any signs of nausea or diarrhea (again, beyond what the sickness is already causing). Although you want to raise the dose of MMS1 to what the child can tolerate, there is a stopping point. Never give the child more than the maximum amounts of MMS1 listed below, which are calculated according to the weight of the child. Please note, the weight scale for MMS1 is calculated differently than in Protocol 1000, because the amounts of MMS1 are significantly higher while on Protocol 2000.

Protocol 2000 for Children Maximum Dosage Guide for MMS1	
Weight	**Drops Per Hour**
10 lbs or less (4.5 kilos or less)	Take no more than 3 drops hourly.
10-20 lbs (5-9 kg)	Take no more than 5 drops hourly.
20-40 lbs (9-18 kg)	Take no more than 5 drops hourly.
40-60 lbs (18-27 kg)	Take no more than 6 drops hourly.
60-80 lbs (27-36 kg)	Take no more than 7 drops hourly.

Protocol 2000 for Children—MMS2 Doses

Protocol 2000 calls for taking MMS2 in capsule form, while also taking MMS1. I do not suggest giving MMS2 to children under 75 lbs. If the child is over 75 lbs and has a life threatening disease you may want to consider giving him/her MMS2, especially if MMS1 is not available. However, do not use MMS2 for children unless the child **knows how to take capsules and can be trusted to swallow it down immediately,** not let it linger in their mouth, not bite down on it, chew it, or break it open in their mouth, as this would not be a pleasant experience. Please **use caution**.

Do not give a child MMS 2 (only for 75 lbs [34 kg] and up) unless you have thoroughly read and studied the instructions in the section on Protocol 2000, page 89, and the section MMS2—Details, page 274, for instructions on how to make MMS2 capsules, and cautions about MMS2 and DMSO.

Protocol 2000 for Children Dosage Guide for MMS2	
Weight	**Size of MMS2 Capsule**
Children under 75 lbs (34 kg)	Do not use MMS2 for children under 75 lbs.
Children 75-100 lbs (34-45 kg) and up	Use a #3 capsule filled to 1/8 full at first, then work up in increments to a 3/4 full capsule.

Protocol 3000 for Children

This is an adaptation of the original Protocol 3000 which can be used for children. The amounts of MMS1 and DMSO used here are the same as in Protocol 3000 for adults. However, it is the method of applying the mixture to a child's skin that is different. The method below is more convenient. Please familiarize yourself with DMSO and how to properly use it before using this protocol. (See Chapter 4 for more details about how to handle DMSO.)

Instructions for Protocol 3000 for Children

Preparation

❑ You will need three spray bottles, preferably either 2 or 4 ounce/60 or 120 ml bottles. Glass spray bottles if you can get them, are best for DMSO. If glass is not available, be sure you get plastic spray bottles that are **compatible** with DMSO. Look for a #1 or #2 inside of a triangle on the bottom of the bottle. This is either PETE or HDPE plastic. (If you cannot find the proper compatible spray bottle for DMSO, it would be best **not** to spray DMSO on but instead pat the DMSO on with your hand.)

❑ Make sure the spray bottles are completely clean.

❑ Clearly **label each bottle** so their contents will not be mistaken.

❑ Prepare the clean, dry bottles as follows:

Bottle #1: Standard **MMS1** spray bottle—10 drops of MMS1 per ounce of water (see page 76).

Bottle #2: Fill the bottle with **DMSO**. You may want to dilute it a little with purified water if the child has sensitive skin. But the stronger the DMSO the better as long as there is absolutely no problem with itching or burning.

Bottle #3: Fill a clean spray bottle with purified water (bottled, distilled or reverse osmosis). **Make sure it is clearly marked as water.**

Applying MMS1/DMSO to the Skin

Before using this protocol, it is best to test the child for any possible allergy to DMSO (see allergy test on page 59). If there are no signs of allergy, before beginning this procedure ask the child to tell you if it hurts, stings, or burns the minute he feels it.

Step 1

Test the Skin

❑ On a bare clean portion of the child's arm, spray one single spray of bottle #3 (water bottle) on an area about the size of your hand.

❑ Then spray one single spray with bottle #1 (MMS1) right on top of the same area.

❑ Immediately spray one single spray with bottle #2 (DMSO), right on top of the same area.

❑ Then take your bare hand and gently rub in the ingredients in a circular motion.

❑ Give it about five minutes to see if there will be any stinging, burning or itching. If there is any of these, spray some more water on the area, and rub it in gently.

❑ If the test does not cause any burning, stinging or itching, proceed to Step 2.

❑ If any burning, stinging or itching persists, then rinse the test area well, add as much as 20% pure water to the DMSO spray bottle and repeat the test on a new area of the skin.

❑ If irritation occurs the second time, dilute the DMSO further. Keep repeating this process until there is no skin irritation.

Step 2

Applying MMS1 and DMSO

❑ Spray a very light spray of water on one of the child's arms on the top side. With your hand gently spread the water in order to dampen the area. Do not use a lot of water, but just enough to make the skin damp.

❑ After applying the water, spray MMS1 on the same area on the top of the arm, and then spray DMSO on top of that. Gently spread the mixture over the area with a bare hand. (Do not use rubber or latex gloves.)

❑ If the skin where you sprayed seems too dry you can add an additional spray of MMS1 and DMSO, and again gently rub it.

❑ After spreading the mixture, allow it to dry on the arm if there is no irritation. Leave it on the skin for several hours before washing.

Step 3

❑ In one hour repeat these same steps on the other arm.

Step 4

❑ Continue with these steps hourly, covering a different area of the body each time. Go to one leg, and then the other leg, and then if everything is ok go to the back, and then the stomach. Be gentle and use plenty of water if needed to avoid pain, itching or burning.

Safety Precautions

I want to emphasis the following, especially when using this procedure for children, to assure there is absolutely no harm done to the child:

- If the MMS1/DMSO mixture burns or irritates the skin, this indicates the DMSO is too strong (various skin types can handle different strengths of DMSO).

- If your DMSO bottle is too strong, keep diluting it with distilled or purified water, up to a total of 50% water until there is no problem with burning or pain.

- If irritation does occur, spray on some more water quickly until the child says there is no more hurt.

- In the case of burning, rinse the DMSO off with lots of plain water (do not use tap water to rinse the skin, in this case, purified water is best). Do not use soap until you have rinsed the area very well, as DMSO can carry small amounts of soap into the skin.

- Rinse your hands well with purified water after applying the MMS1 and DMSO.

Protocol 6 and 6 for Children

Protocol 6 and 6 consists of two 6-drop doses of MMS1 taken separately, one hour apart. This protocol is particularly effective for colds, flu, pains, allergies and other sicknesses that seem to just be starting. It is helpful for a wide range of things. See page 169 for more details and full instructions on Protocol 6 and 6; however, adjust the dosage for children according to the chart below.

Protocol 6 and 6 for Children	
Weight	MMS1 Drops Per Hour
Babies 12 lbs (5.5 kg) and less	1 and 1 drop dose
Children 12-24 lbs (5.5-11 kg)	2 and 2 drop dose
Children 25-49 lbs (11-23 kg)	3 and 3 drop dose
Children 50-74 lbs (23-34 kg)	4 and 4 drop dose
Children 75-100 lbs (34-45 kg)	5 and 5 drop dose
People 100-lbs and up. (45-kg and up)	6 and 6 drop dose

MMS1/DMSO Patch Protocol for Babies, Children and People with Sensitive Skin

Please read and have a good understanding of the instructions for the standard MMS1/DMSO Patch Protocol on page 135. This is basically the same procedure but the amounts of MMS1 drops/water and the timing for applying the patch is adjusted to accommodate babies, children and people with sensitive skin.

❑ Apply to clean skin. Start with 5 drops of MMS1 (activated MMS), add 5 drops of DMSO and 10 additional drops of water to dilute the solution.

❑ For the very first application do not apply the patch for more than five minutes.

❑ When the patch is removed take note if there is irritation. If there is no irritation after five minutes with the first patch, in two hours apply another patch. This time you can leave it on for 15 minutes.

❑ If there is no skin irritation or burning on the next 15-minute application it is OK to continue with these applications.

❑ If at any time there is skin irritation or burning, then double the additional amount of water beyond what was used on the last application.

Daily MMS1 Maintenance Dose for Children

Children, as a rule, are exposed to a wide variety of toxins throughout the day; they play on the floor or in the dirt, put dirty hands into their mouths, etc. This is one of many reasons, why a daily MMS1 maintenance dose may be important for your child. For full details on the MMS1 Maintenance Dose (for adults and children), please see pages 200-201.

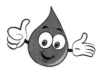

Child Free of Frequent Illness: My son (4 years old) suffered with asthma and other chronic bronchial problems, falling sick on an average of every two weeks for over two years. Since discovering MMS, he is not only free from respiratory problems, but when other things are "going around" he remains healthy thanks to a daily MMS1 maintenance dose. –Veronica, Mexico

How to Adjust Supporting Protocols and Additional Protocols for Children

The following charts explain how to adjust all other Protocols for children.

Babies 12 lbs (5.5 kg) and Less	
Protocol	**Dosage**
Bag Treatment	Do not use.
Baths and Foot Baths	Use 1/4 number of drops of adult dose —page 143.
Black Widow Bite	Same as adults —page 217.
Brown Recluse Spider Bite	Same as adults —page 213.
Burns	Same as adults —page 245.
Enema	Use 1/4 number of drops of adult dose —page 148.
Eyes/Ears/Nose	Use 1/8 drop of MMS1 per ounce of distilled water for the eyes; and 1/4 drop per ounce of distilled water for the ears and nose — page 136.
Food Poisoning	Use 1/4 number of drops of adult dose —page 223.
Mold/Fungus	Use 1/8 tsp clay doses/adjust MMS1 to weight—page 99.
Heart Attacks	Use 1/8 the drops and 1/8 the DMSO an adult would use (page 236). Also do the 6 and 6 but for children of this weight, which is actually 1 and 1 (page 265).
Indian Herb	Do not use.
Mouth and Teeth	Use 1 drop of MMS1 per ounce of water —page 73.
Protocol 4000	Do not use for babies.
Spray Bottle	Use 3 drops MMS1 per ounce of water —page 76.
Strokes	Use 1/8 the drops and 1/8 the DMSO an adult would use (page 227). Also do Protocol 6 and 6 for babies, which would actually be 1 and 1 (page 265).

Children 12-24 lbs (5.5-11 kg)	
Protocol	Dosage
Bag Treatment	Do not use.
Baths and Foot Baths	Use 1/4 number of drops of adult dose —page 143.
Black Widow Bite	Same as adults —page 217.
Brown Recluse Spider Bite	Same as adults —page 213.
Burns	Same as adults —page 245.
Enema	Use 1/4 number of drops of adult dose —page 148.
Eyes/Ears/Nose	Use 1/8 drop of MMS1 per ounce of distilled water for eyes and 1/2 drop of MMS1 per ounce of distilled water for ears and nose —page 136.
Food Poisoning	Use 1/4 number of drops of adult dose —page 223.
Mold/Fungus	Use 1/4 tsp clay doses/adjust MMS1 to weight—page 99.
Heart Attacks	Use 1/8 the drops and 1/8 the DMSO an adult would use (page 236). Also do the 6 and 6 but for children of this weight, which is actually 2 and 2 (page 265).
Indian Herb	Do not use.
Mouth and Teeth	Use 1 drop of MMS1 per ounce of water —page 73.
Protocol 4000	Do not use for a child of this weight.
Spray Bottle	Use 3 drops MMS1 per ounce of water —page 76.
Strokes	Use 1/8 the drops and 1/8 the DMSO an adult would use (page 227). Also do Protocol 6 and 6, but for children of this weight it would be 2 and 2 (page 265).

Children 25-49 lbs (11-23 kg)	
Protocol	**Dosage**
Bag Treatment	Do not use.
Baths and Foot Baths	Use 1/4 number of drops of adult dose —page 143.
Black Widow Bite	Same as adults —page 217.
Brown Recluse Spider Bite	Same as adults —page 213.
Burns	Same as adults —page 245.
Enema	Use 1/4 number of drops of adult dose —page 148.
Eyes/Ears/Nose	Use 1/4 drop of MMS1 in each ounce of water for eyes and 1/2 drop of MMS1 per ounce of water for ears and nose —page 136.
Food Poisoning	Use 1/4 number of drops of adult dose —page 223.
Mold/Fungus	Use 1/2 tsp clay doses/adjust MMS1 to weight—page 99.
Heart Attacks	Use 1/4 the drops and 1/4 the DMSO that an adult would use (page 236). Also do Protocol 6 and 6 but for children of this weight it is actually 3 and 3 (page 265).
Indian Herb	Do not use.
Mouth and Teeth	Use 1 drop of MMS1 per ounce of water —page 73.
Protocol 4000	Do not use for a child of this weight.
Spray Bottle	Use 5 drops MMS1 per ounce of water —page 76.
Strokes	Use 1/4 the drops and 1/4 the DMSO an adult would use (page 227). Also do Protocol 6 and 6, but for children of this weight it would be 3 and 3 (page 265).

| Children 50-74 lbs (23-34 kg) ||
Protocol	Dosage
Bag Treatment	Use 1/2 the number of drops an adult would use —page 156.
Baths and Foot Baths	Use 1/2 number of drops of adult dose —page 143.
Black Widow Bite	Same as adults —page 217.
Brown Recluse Spider Bite	Same as adults —page 213.
Burns	Same as adults —page 245.
Enema	Use 1/2 number of drops of adult dose —page 148.
Eyes/Ears/Nose	Use 1/4 drop of MMS1 in each ounce of water for eyes and 1/2 drop of MMS1 per ounce of water for ears and nose —page 136.
Food Poisoning	Use 3/4 number of drops of adult dose —page 223.
Mold/Fungus	Use 3/4 tsp clay doses/adjust MMS1 to weight—page 99.
Heart Attacks	Use 1/2 the drops and 1/2 the DMSO that an adult would use (page 236). Also do Protocol 6 and 6, but for children of this weight it is actually 4 and 4 (page 265).
Indian Herb	Follow the instructions that come with the Indian Herb—page 165.
Mouth and Teeth	Use 2 drop of MMS1 per ounce of water —page 73.
Protocol 4000	Do not use for a child of this weight.
Spray Bottle	Use 10 drops MMS1 per ounce of water —page 76.
Strokes	Use 1/2 the drops and 1/2 the DMSO an adult would use (page 227). Also do Protocol 6 and 6, but for children of this weight it would be 4 and 4 (page 265).

Children 75-100 lbs (34-45 kg)	
Protocol	Dosage
Bag Treatment	Use 1/2 the number of drops an adult would use —page 156.
Baths and Foot Baths	Use the same number of drops that an adult would use —page 143.
Black Widow Bite	Same as adults —page 217.
Brown Recluse Spider Bite	Same as adults —page 213.
Burns	Same as adults —page 245.
Enema	Use the same number of drops an adult would use —page 148.
Eyes/Ears/Nose	Use 1/4 drop of MMS1 per ounce of water for eyes and 1 drop of MMS1 per ounce of water for ears and nose —page 136.
Food Poisoning	Same as adults —page 223.
Mold/Fungus	Use 1 tsp clay doses/adjust MMS1 to weight—page 99.
Heart Attacks	Use MMS1 and DMSO the same as adults (page 236). Also do Protocol 6 and 6, but for children of this weight it is actually 5 and 5 (page 265).
Indian Herb	Follow the instructions that come with the Indian Herb.—page 165.
Mouth and Teeth	Use 2.5 drops of MMS1 per ounce of water —page 73.
Protocol 4000	Use a size 4 capsule filled to 1/4 at first and then work up to a 3/4 full capsule in two days and thereafter—page 171.
Spray Bottle	Use 10 drops MMS1 per ounce of water —page 76.
Strokes	Use 3/4 the drops and 3/4 the DMSO an adult would use (page 227). Also do Protocol 6 and 6, but for children of this weight it would be 5 and 5 (page 265).

Anal Fistula: I'm writing...to say you saved my brother. This year in May my brother suffered from anal fistula for the fourth time. He has been suffering from anal fistula since 2001. The fourth time was this year in May and he was really sick, he couldn't walk, his legs hurt, his feet hurt and he was really worried, he said he never felt so bad in his whole life. I started treating him with the protocol 1000, that is 3 activated drops of MMS every hour and I prepared a spray bottle with 40 activated drops of MMS to spray on the affected area continuously every time it dried up. After taking MMS for one day his legs and feet started feeling better and he could stand up straight and walk around slowly. Day three he didn't feel any pain at all and we were all happy about it. Day four he went shopping with his wife. He was really ok. Day five he went back to work, he said he felt stronger than ever, full of energy. Just like me he is now taking 6 drops of activated drops of MMS every day for maintenance. He told me that now he was doing things he couldn't do before because his back was hurting as he was moving or lifting objects around. Now he is a healthy person. —Vincent, Italy

Diabetes: I brought my friend with diabetes over and treated him every hour for five or six hours because his blood sugar was close to 500. His blood sugar went down to 91 in those short hours. FACT! —C.P. United States

Chapter 14

Additional Important Information

Biofilms

A biofilm is a thin resistant layer of microorganisms that form on and coat wet surfaces. They are well-organized colonies of bacteria clustered together to form micro-colonies. Biofilms can be formed by a single bacterial species, but biofilms more often consist of many species of bacteria, as well as fungi, algae, protozoa, debris, and corrosion products. Essentially, a biofilm may form on any surface exposed to bacteria and some amount of water. In industry biofilms form in many places such as in water pipes, water tanks and cooling towers. Biofilms can also form in or on the human body and thus are responsible for many diseases.

When these colonies of bacteria cluster together, they secrete a special mucus that cements them together in a film-like concoction. When this happens other pathogens can hide in them and beneath them. Biofilms can make healing in the body more difficult or often impossible. They are highly resistant to antibiotics. Medical drugs seem to have little, if any, effect on them. However, MMS can overcome biofilm, both inside and outside the body.

If you have been taking MMS and are improving, but at a very slow rate, it may be an indication that you have biofilm somewhere in your system. The answer is to simply continue on the protocol until you are feeling well. This could be anywhere from a few days to a few weeks and in some cases a few months, before the biofilm is totally killed. Keep at it until you are feeling good.

If you have been taking MMS with no problem, and all of a sudden at the same dosage you experience a significant Herxhiemer reaction, you have probably broken through a biofilm. The die-off of the pathogens hits you in one big burst, which causes a Herxheimer reaction. The good news is, you are then able to get rid of the toxins that have been causing you problems and your body can heal.

Biofilms on the outside of the body normally only happen in sores or wounds where there is continuous moisture. When they are present in the sore or wound they often cause healing to take much longer or prevent healing altogether. For this, I suggest using the MMS1 spray bottle as directed on page 76. In situations where the biofilm seems to be resistant to the normal strength spray bottle of 10 drops of MMS1 per 1 ounce (30 ml) of water, in other words, the sore or wound is not healing, I suggest you increase the amount of drops in the spray bottle. First try putting 20 drops of MMS1 per 1 ounce (30 ml) of water in the bottle. If you still do not see good results with 20 drops per ounce, increase the drops in the spray bottle in increments. You can go up to 50 MMS1 drops per ounce (30 ml) of water, if you feel it's needed.

MMS2—Details

MMS2, calcium hypochlorite, is sometimes known as Pool Shock. It is sold in pool stores and grocery stores throughout the world. As long as it is for swimming pools, manufacturers cannot put bad things in the pools that would hurt swimmers, and thus cannot put harmful things in the calcium hypochlorite. The package will say it contains somewhere from 45% to 85% available chlorine. **This is not true.** As long as you have **calcium** hypochlorite (not **sodium** hypochlorite, which does produce chlorine) there is no available chlorine. When calcium hypochlorite is dissolved in water it turns into **hypochlorous acid (HOCl)** and there is no chlorine available. HOCl is the same acid that your body naturally generates to kill disease and destroy poisons. When you take MMS2, you are giving your body more of its own ammunition against disease. The microorganisms in a swimming pool are killed by the calcium hypochlorite which is turned into HOCl. Manufacturers only say there is "available chlorine" in order to make the calcium hypochlorite sell, as many in the world unfortunately still think that chlorine is a safe and effective product for killing microorganisms—and it is a common mistake to mix up these terms. Chlorine, which is **sodium** hypochlorite, will kill microorganisms, but it also is harmful to the human body. **Calcium** hypochlorite, which when added to water produces hypochlorous acid, will also kill microorganisms, but it is not harmful to the human body and does not contain the chemical "chlorine".

Instructions

Step 1

❏ Purchase calcium hypochlorite from pool stores, chemical supply stores, grocery stores, and in some countries, it can even be found in department stores.

Step 2

❏ Purchase some empty gel or vegetable capsules, size #1 or #0. If you cannot find these, purchase a regular bottle of some type of vitamin capsules in one of these same sizes. Empty the capsules by pulling them apart. (It is best to purchase clear/transparent capsules. Some capsules come in colors, and the *color (dye)* can sometimes be harmful.)

Step 3

❑ Partially fill the capsules with the calcium hypochlorite granules. Do not try to grind the granules finer. Just use the granules as they are. Allow them to fall loosely into the capsules without packing them down. Always start low in the amount you add to your capsule and increase your doses gradually. When the capsules are pulled apart, one side is always larger than the other side. Fill the larger side. Then put the smaller side on and be sure you push it down securely in place.

❑ For size #1 capsules, start by filling a capsule 1/8 full. Then increase the amount slowly over several days, until you reach a full size #1 capsule.

❑ For #0 size capsules start by filling a capsule 1/16 full. Increase the amount slowly over several days. Do not fill a #0 size capsule more than 3/4 full.

Step 4

❑ Always take MMS2 capsules two hours apart.

❑ Always drink the first MMS2 capsule down with 1 full cup (8 ounces/240 ml) of water. With each capsule after that, drink at least 1/2 cup (4 ounces/120 ml) of water, but drink more if you need it.

❑ When you begin taking these capsules, start with taking one capsule at the lowest dose. Two hours later take another capsule also at the lowest dose.

❑ Then two hours later, on the third capsule increase the amount of MMS2 in the capsule a little bit, and take it. Two hours later, take the fourth capsule with the same amount of MMS2 you put in the third capsule.

❑ If there are no problems after taking these 4 capsules, then continue increasing the amount of MMS2 in your capsules until you reach the maximum size dose. Stick with that as your standard MMS2 dose for the duration of time you are taking MMS2. In case of nausea or diarrhea reduce the amount of calcium hypochlorite in each capsule by 50%. When these symptoms subside, slowly increase the amount to the suggested doses given above.

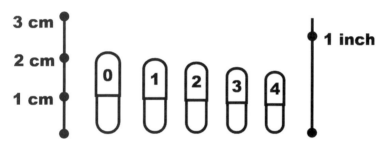

Notes

➤ *If at any time while increasing the amount of MMS2 in these capsules you feel signs of a Herxheimer reaction coming on, slow down on the rate at which you increase the amount of powder in the capsule. It is not a race. If you cannot increase to the maximum size dose, stick with the size dose you are comfortable with. Follow the Three Golden Rules.*

➤ *If you have purchased MMS2 capsules already made up, you may need to open the capsules and empty out some of the powder in order to follow the above instructions.*

> *These are the general guidelines for making MMS2 capsules. See Protocol 2000 or Protocol 4000 for specific instructions on dosing with MMS2.*

> **It is important to never take a dose containing an MMS2 capsule and DMSO at the same time.** *See pages 23-24 for the full warning on this.*

Testing to See if Liquids are Compatible with MMS1

Anytime we use a liquid other than water to make our MMS1 dose, we need to know that the liquid does not cancel out the effectiveness of MMS1. This means that the liquid is *compatible* with MMS1. If the MMS1 is destroyed or nearly destroyed by the liquid, we then say the liquid is *not compatible* with MMS1. You can determine if a liquid is compatible with MMS1, by measuring the parts per million of MMS1 in the liquid. This should be done both immediately upon making an MMS1 dose and again after one hour by measuring the same dose. If the strength has not deteriorated beyond a certain amount in one hour we can say the liquid is compatible with MMS1.

Parts per million is one way of expressing very dilute concentrations of substances. Just as *per cent* means out of a hundred, so *parts per million,* or ppm, means out of a million. Parts per million often describes the concentration of something in water or liquid. So if you have 25 ppm of MMS1 in half a cup (4 ounces/120 ml) of water, this means if the half cup of water were divided into a million parts, only 25 of those million parts would be MMS1.

The active ingredient in MMS1 is chlorine dioxide. There are test strips manufactured by LaMotte Company that we can use for the purpose of determining the concentration (ppm) of chlorine dioxide in an MMS1 dose. The strips are dipped into the solution and the color that the strip turns tells us how many parts per million (ppm) of chlorine dioxide are in the solution. If you want to use a liquid other than water for your MMS1 dose but, you are not sure if it will cancel out the effectiveness of MMS1, then follow the instructions below to test for compatibility.

The LaMotte High Range Chlorine Dioxide Test Strips read from 0 to 500 ppm. Directions on the bottle may confuse you a little bit as it only mentions in one place that the strip is for the purpose of testing ppm. In any case, follow the instructions on the bottle. Be sure to do the testing where there is plenty of light (not in dim light), so you can evaluate the colors accurately.

Instructions

Step 1

❑ Measure out 1/2 cup (4 ounces/120 ml) of any liquid that you want to test to see if you can use that liquid for taking a dose of MMS1. All teas, juices, soft drinks and other liquids other than what has been mentioned in this book as compatible with MMS1, should be tested.

❑ Mix up a 3-drop dose of MMS1 and pour it into the 4 ounces/120 ml of liquid that you have just prepared. Stir well to evenly distribute the chlorine dioxide in the liquid.

Step 2

❑ Remove a single test strip from the LaMotte container and dip it into the 4 ounces of liquid containing your 3-drop properly prepared dose. (Do not move the strip around while in the liquid.)

❑ Count two seconds using the "one one-thousand, two one-thousand" method, then remove the strip from the liquid. (Do not flick any of the liquid off the strip when you take it out.) Do a similar count up to ten and then check the color on the strip with the color chart on the side of the LaMotte container. When you use 3 MMS1 drops in 4 ounces/120 ml of liquid, your number as indicated by the color on the strip, should be between 25 and 50.

Step 3

❑ Cover and set aside your liquid (out of the light) with the 3 drops of MMS1 and wait one hour.

Step 4

❑ After one hour, do the same test over again with the same liquid, but with a new test strip. The number indicated by the color on the strip as compared to the color chart should again be between 25 and 50, and if it is, your liquid is compatible with MMS1.

❑ If the reading on the strip goes down after one hour, this means in an hour the MMS in the liquid has lost some potency. If it hasn't gone down too much, (the strip should not read less than about 20 when compared to the color chart), you could still use that type of liquid providing every time you drink your dose, you take it immediately after putting the MMS1 in. (As a rule, you should always take your MMS1 dose within a minute of mixing it up.)

Notes

➤ *It is important to keep the bottle of your test strips tightly capped at all times when not in use. This will keep moisture out, which can affect the readings.*

➤ *You can cut the strips lengthwise to get 100 strips instead of 50.*

➤ *When cutting or handling the strips, be sure to not touch the strip's pad with your fingers, or your readings may not be accurate.*

High Range Chlorine Dioxide Test Strips (code #3002) made by LaMotte are available on the market with two different labels, although both are the same product. (In any case, be sure to check the code number.) Both labels show the same measuring color chart on the outside of the container.

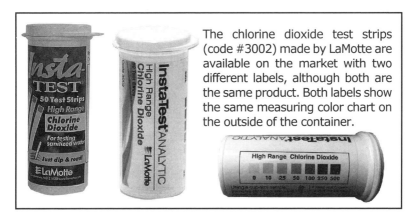

The chlorine dioxide test strips (code #3002) made by LaMotte are available on the market with two different labels, although both are the same product. Both labels show the same measuring color chart on the outside of the container.

Available over the internet at:

➤ LaMotte Company:

   http://www.lamotte.com/en/browse/3002.html

(Go to this webpage, choose the distributor nearest you and check with them to make sure they carry the test strips.)

> ➤ Also available at:

https://www.amazon.com
(Search for LaMotte 3002.)

Pain Relief

Pain in the body can be for many varied reasons. Some-times it is due to a build-up of toxins stored in the joints. MMS has proven to eliminate pain in a significant number of cases. Although it sounds too good to be true, we have many reports from people who have suffered from pain for many years and found relief with two simple doses of MMS1 (Protocol 6 and 6). However, there are other pains in the back, head, neck, and in joints of the body that are often caused by the muscles pulling against one another. This can cause extreme pain. In this case, MMS may not relieve the pain and I suggest you check out a book called *Pain Free* by Pete Egoscue. Pete has over 30 clinics worldwide and his method has helped thousands of people relieve pain not caused directly by disease.

Pain in the neck, back, hands, knees and other joints can cause tremendous problems. When the muscles pull against one another they can cause the cartilage to disappear from your joints. Medical doctors will tell you it cannot be repaired. I beg to differ. The book *Pain Free* shows you simple exercises, which I call "relax-a-cisers." With these simple (but possibly awkward to the beginner) exercise positions, you relax your muscles to the point that they move away from one another. They get un-stuck and therefore this action relieves the pain you are experiencing.

It has been reported that millions of people have avoided operations and replacement of joints merely by following the exercises taught by Pete Egoscue in his clinics and books. If you have pain of this kind, it will be worth your while to obtain this information and follow the procedures. Normally pain is gone in a few weeks or less.

Parasites

There is an old saying that seems to prove true most of the time, and that is, "we need to have a balance in all things". Because someone has discovered some parasites in their body is not a reason to jump right into harsh poisonous treatments to expel them all. Let me explain.

First, I want to point out that this is not by any means meant to be all comprehensive on the theme of parasites. This is a vast subject and there can be a wide variety of reasons why parasites can cause problems in the human body. This information is food for thought, as well as some pointers on where to get started when trying to rid (or reduce) the body of unwanted parasites.

There are many types of parasites, and it might surprise some people to discover that not all parasites are bad, and expelling them from the body is not always the best thing to do. There are quite a few books available today pointing out that the human body needs parasites. Parasites do not **always** come from eating the wrong thing, or from walking through the woods, or through the grass, or walking along the sea shore in bare feet. Parasites show up in various parts of the body when needed because of an existing bad condition. Parasites do not eat healthy flesh or tissues. They eat dying and rotten tissues and other microorganisms that may be dead. Normally, they are not there to hurt the area, but rather to *clean up* the mess. They are often one of the body's last stands against a bad problem that is hurting the body.

Many parasites are symbiotic. (Interaction between two different organisms living in close physical association, typically to the advantage of both.) Parasites often come from within our bodies, and, as I mentioned above, not always from outside the body. We get rid of them by restoring health to the body, not by using various poisons to kill them. Poisons for parasites are also poisons for us and they do a certain amount of damage to our bodies. It is somewhat like using chemotherapy. Allopathic medicine advocates very harmful poisons to try to kill cancer before the cancer kills the body. At least that is the theory, and using poisons to kill parasites is similar. I believe that first using MMS1 to kill the pathogens and remove the heavy metals and toxins that cause disease is the best way to go. MMS1 is able to correct the cause of disease and then the body can repair itself and parasites are likely to be expelled in the process as well. Do as much good as you can with MMS1 and then consider what is necessary to further handle the parasites if needed.

The first step would be to follow the protocols in this book. These protocols have overcome thousands of unhealthy conditions. Start at the beginning with the Starting Procedure and follow through as the Health Recovery Plan indicates. Once your body has healed, then the parasites—not having dead flesh or toxins to feed on—will die off, then the body can expel worms and parasites naturally through the bowels if they are functioning properly.

Now, having said all that, remember what I said about balance. There are times when a person can have too many parasites. I'm not saying there is never a need to expel them. There are many reasons, too many to name here, why parasites may get out of hand. But briefly, as I said, many parasites are symbiotic—many come from within our body, **but not all**. There is no doubt that some enter the body in our food and through other ways. Thankfully, nature has provided ways for handling these things if everything is working properly in the body. When stomach acid is normal for example, this destroys most parasites and/or parasite eggs that enter the body through food. Regular bowel movements also keep things moving and parasite larva goes through before it has a chance to latch on to the colon and hatch. When one gets drastically constipated and things get backed up, it's another story. Some suggest that a highly nutritious diet will keep parasites at bay. So there are many whys and wherefores as to why some people have a high amount of parasites and others do not.

In any case, if the parasites get too far out of balance, large quantities of parasites must be addressed directly. If a person has healed their body from disease or conditions that brought on parasites to *clean things up*, but an imbalance of parasites persists, then taking extra steps to rid the body of parasites is necessary. I suggest more natural ways to accomplish this, rather than using pharmaceutical drugs.

Most health food stores have various natural remedies for killing or balancing parasites in the body. Likewise, there are many herbs and foods in nature that accomplish this purpose if taken correctly. Some researchers have shown that parasites are particularly vulnerable to a variety of herbs which are lethal only to them. Investigate and find out what is common in your country and location.

Look up Dr. Hulda Clark's *Herbal Parasite Cleanse for Beginners* on the internet:

http://www.drclark.net/cleanses/beginners/herbal-parasite-cleanse/parasite-chart-for-adults

In addition, there are those who use electrical frequencies to kill parasites and that sometimes is beneficial without hurting the body. I believe that the electric current frequency machines work well, but in thousands of cases I have personally not found many folks that really needed to destroy their parasites with the electric frequency machine. But, in the case where it is needed, I would recommend Pavel's electronic zapper machine. For information go to:

www.ravozapper.com

I should also mention that Pavel's machine can be adjusted to kill pathogens which cause a wide variety of diseases other than parasites, thus restoring health just like MMS.

Nature provides many things within the body which we have not learned to use. Modern science for the most part has not tried to learn these things. When a body dies if it is put in a completely sterile room where there are no germs or pathogens or worms, within a few hours the body will be riddled with parasitic worms which will, in a few days, destroy the body completely except for the skeleton. All those worms came from within the body, not from walking through the woods. We cheat nature of its job by taking a corpse to the mortuary and embalming it with a poison that preserves it and kills the worms that would otherwise return it to dust. Nature provides for decomposing the body back to nature once it dies and nature provides parasites (of which many are really symbiotic organisms) that help the body to overcome some extremely bad conditions.

Note: *Some people are of the opinion that there is a connection between autism, parasites and vaccines. My suspicion is that the vaccines confuse the natural parasites and also create a more toxic environment that the para-*

sites try to clean up. They may go overboard and repro-
duce to the point of causing a problem in the person and
thereby contribute to the symptoms of autism. By detoxing
the body and reducing the parasite population, thousands
of children with autism have shown significant improve-
ments. Check out Kerri Rivera's book, Healing the Symp-
toms known as Autism.

Water Purification with MMS

MMS1 for water purification: To treat plain clear water
that you feel should be purified to kill disease pathogens,
such as tap water from your faucet, I suggest adding 8
drops of MMS1 (activated MMS—use 50% citric acid or
4% HCl) per gallon of water (or 4 liters/4 quarts). Count
30 seconds for the drops to activate then put the mixture
into a gallon of water. Mix thoroughly, cover and wait for
at least one hour before use. Keep in mind MMS1 does not
kill the chlorine or the fluoride in your water but it will kill
diseases. For smaller quantities of water, use less drops.
For 1 quart (or liter) use 2 drops of MMS1.

Turpid (cloudy) water requires more MMS1. If you have a
slight bit of turbidity, use 12 drops of activated MMS1 per
gallon. A higher amount of turbidity requires higher
amounts of MMS. Use 12 to 24 of MMS1 drops or even
more drops for river water. This is something you will
have to evaluate and do your best to get it right. In this
case, it is always best to error on the side of too many
drops than not enough. A slightly bad taste resulting from
the MMS1 (if you have to go higher) will not hurt you.

MMS2 for water purification: Water can be purified
using MMS2 equally as well as MMS1. (Like MMS1, MMS2
does not kill the chlorine or the fluoride in your water but
it will kill diseases.) Both MMS1 and MMS2 are used
throughout the world to purify water in public water

systems. One #1 size capsule (see page 46 for capsule size) filled 1/2 full of calcium hypochlorite (MMS2) can be used to purify one gallon of normal appearing clear water. I have found that using gelatin or vegetable capsules is a very convenient method of measuring small amounts of powdered MMS2. Do not pack tightly or compress the MMS2 in the capsule, but loosely fill the capsule to 1/2 full. Open the capsule and pour the powder from the capsule into the water. Stir well until dissolved, cover and wait two hours before use.

Turbid (cloudy) water requires more MMS2. If you have a slight bit of turbidity, use a full #1 size capsule of MMS2. In the case of more turbidity, you can use up to 2 full size #1 capsules of MMS2 for a gallon of water. Use 1 to 3 capsules for river water. Again this is something you will have to evaluate. In this case of purifying questionable water, it is always best to error on the side of too much MMS2 rather than not enough. You may alter the taste of the water with 3 capsules, but that would be a lot better than getting sick from the water. Three capsules of MMS2 in a gallon of water will not hurt you even if it tastes a little bad.

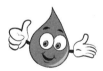

Animal cure: My dog had a bad skin disease that left him with no hair only raw skin. Having MMS in my cupboard, I decided to try it...Within two weeks all his hair had grown back plus he has no itch. I started giving him three drops twice a day and increased it by one, so he has been on four drops for the second week. He has fully recovered with great health. I put the mixture in his meat and he ate it all. We were so overwhelmed my husband said if it grew hair back on my dog why wouldn't it grow my hair back. So my husband is on it now. —Didi, Australia

Chapter 15

Animals

Protocol for Animals

All of the protocols in this book can be applied to most animals (there are some variations for ruminants, see page 290) from hamsters to dogs and cats, to horses, and other large animals. This chapter on animals is not meant to be comprehensive by any means. Time and space do not permit at the time of this writing. However, I do want to give you some general guidelines and rules for animals, which if followed should allow you to handle most of their diseases and health problems.

As mentioned in the Preface of this book, those of you who have read my previous writings on MMS may notice some variations here to what I've published in the past. For animals, as with humans, through on-going use of MMS we have learned new things. It has become more and more obvious that animals and humans react to the healing benefits of MMS in similar ways.

Please read this entire animal chapter as it contains important details you will need to know in order to help your animal recover health. Basically all the same rules apply for animals as with people when using MMS. That is, if the animal seems to get better with what you are doing, keep up with what you are doing. Do not change anything. If the animal seems to get sicker with MMS, such as having diarrhea or vomiting, then reduce the dosage you are giving by one half, but do not stop. If you do not see positive results of any kind within about two days, you would then go to the next level of protocol. **With animals, I suggest less waiting time** than with people before going to the next level of the protocol, because normally animals respond (heal) faster than humans. For the most part you can help an animal with MMS pretty much the same as a human. If you have read and carefully studied this book, the same rules and principles apply, with some minor adjustments.

➤ Ruminants (e.g., cows, sheep, goats, etc.) are different than humans, cats, dogs, etc., in that they have a four-compartment stomach. I do not have a great deal of personal experience with these animals, although feedback I have received from those heavily involved with ruminants suggests the following:

These animals are able to take oral doses of MMS1, as long as it is activated with HCl (hydrochloric acid) and not citric acid. Citric acid has been known to cause problems for ruminants. So if using oral doses of MMS1 for a ruminant, use 4% HCl as the activator, or give oral doses of CDS. In addition, a variation of CDS known as CDI (Chlorine Dioxide Injectable) has also been used successfully with these animals. (For more information on CDI, see books from Andreas Kalcker.) Both oral dosing with MMS1 and CDS, and injections with CDI have been successful. We will learn more as time passes, but this has been working so far.

➤ **Horses and some other animals cannot vomit so be careful to not give your animal, especially a horse, too much MMS,** because making a horse sick is more dangerous than making someone sick who can vomit (because vomiting is the body's way of getting rid of unwanted things, poisons, etc.). However, **horses respond to MMS quickly,** usually more quickly than people and I have seen a horse overcome a cold using MMS1 in half an hour. Expect most animals to respond quickly.

Oral Dosages of MMS for Animals

All oral doses of MMS for animals must be calculated according to the weight of the animal. See the charts on pages 301-302.

General Malaise/Sickness

If your animal is not well, and the animal has not been diagnosed with any particular disease (i.e., cancer, etc.) I suggest trying Protocol 6 and 6 first, as per the instructions below.

Protocol 6 and 6 for Animals

Step 1

❑ Give Protocol 6 and 6, **but be sure the amount of MMS is adjusted for the weight of the animal,** as per the chart on page 302. For Protocol 6 and 6 please refer to Column 5 on the chart. Give the animal the first dose (according to the animal's weight), then wait one hour and give your animal a second dose of the same amount.

Step 2

❑ If the animal is well after you have given Protocol 6 and 6 (Step 1 above), the animal can go on the daily maintenance dosage.

Step 3

❑ If however the animal has improved some, or even a lot with one 6 and 6 procedure, but is not all the way well yet, then follow the golden rule that says if things are improving do not change anything—keep doing what you are doing. (See Three Golden Rules for Animals page 305.) In this case however, do not continue with 6-drop doses *every hour*, but after the first 6 and 6 procedure, wait *four* hours, and give the animal another 6 and 6 dosage (remember, these 2 doses are given one hour apart and adjusted for the weight of the animal as per the chart page 302).

❑ If the animal continues to show improvement but is not fully recovered, give 6 and 6 in the morning and 6 and 6 in the evening, as long as the animal is improving, until well. On the other hand, if the animal is no longer improving from the 6 and 6 protocol, and is still sick, then it is time to start him/her on the Health Recovery Plan (HRP) starting with the Starting Procedure and hourly doses.

Note: *The above instructions are a slight variation from Protocol 6 and 6 for humans and moving into hourly doses if two 6-drop doses did not bring recovery. It can sometimes be quite an effort to give an animal an hourly dose. The most important thing is to follow the Three Golden Rules for Animals (see page 305), if you see progress keep doing what is working, and if not, move on to the Health Recovery Plan.*

Step 4

❑ In the case where you give an animal Protocol 6 and 6 one time and they do not show **any** signs of improvement, move right on to the Starting Procedure followed by Protocol 1000 and continue on with the

Health Recovery Plan if needed. Again, remember, all doses for your animal must be adjusted according to the weight, see charts on pages 301-302.

If the Animal Has Been Diagnosed With a Particular Disease

Step 1

❑ If your animal has been diagnosed with a specific disease, such as pneumonia or cancer or any other disease, you will need to begin the Starting Procedure. See Column 1 of the chart on page 301.

Step 2

❑ After completing the Starting Procedure, move on to Protocol 1000 and progress up through Protocol 1000 Plus, 2000, and 3000 according to the Health Recovery Plan as described in this book (see Chapter 5), and the Three Golden Rules for Animals (page 305).

Calculating Doses

The size of the dose should always be determined by the weight of the animal. On pages 301-302 you will find charts to help you determine proper dosages for animals. Please read these charts carefully, as they show the amounts for each animal according to weight. Be attentive to the changes. Follow the guidelines below.

Making Up Less Than 1-Drop Doses: On the chart on page 301, you will note it is sometimes necessary to use a *fraction of a drop* of MMS1 for an animal's dose. This is especially true for smaller animals. In order to make up a fraction of a drop for animals, always activate 1 drop of MMS, count 30 seconds, then add 1 ounce (30 ml) of water. Any amount of water taken out of that 1 ounce of water with 1 drop of MMS1 in it, will always be a fraction of a single drop. For example, if you took 15 milliliters out of that 1 ounce of MMS1 solution you would have 1/2 of a drop of MMS1.

➤ In order to calculate a fraction of a drop you will need the following: A milliliter syringe (a 10 ml syringe works well), and a 1 ounce glass (a shot glass works well). If a 1 ounce shot glass is not available you can improvise. In the clean dry glass activate 1 drop of MMS—count 30 seconds—add 1 ounce (30 ml) of water. To get various fractions of a drop **from this mixture,** take out the amounts of liquid from the 1 ounce (30 ml) solution of MMS1 as shown on the chart below. All calculations on this chart are rounded off to the closest milliliter.

Calculating Fractions of a Drop of MMS1	
Fractions of a Drop	**Liquid to Take From the 1 oz Glass**
1/32nd of a drop	take out 1 ml
1/16th of a drop	take out 2 ml
1/8th of a drop	take out 4 ml
1/4th of a drop	take out 8 ml
1/2 of a drop	take out 15 ml
3/4th of a drop	take out 23 ml
The liquid that is removed from the 1 ounce (30 ml) glass is what you use for the dose. It should be added to more water according to your animal's need.	

Adding water to the animal's dose: Never give an animal MMS1 (activated MMS) without adding the neces-sary water. Each animal is different and will need a different amount of water for its doses. Evaluate your animal carefully. Determine what is a normal drink of water for that animal. According to many experts, an animal needs 1 ounce of water a day for each pound of body weight. (If you are not confident with this figure, you can research further on the internet. Put in a Google search "water required for my animal" and put the type of animal.)

➤ Once you determine the proper daily amount of water your animal needs, I suggest that you use one half of this daily amount of water for its doses of MMS. In other words, take one half of the daily amount of water and divide that by 8 to determine the amount of water you should use for each hourly dose of MMS. For example, if an animal requires 1 liter of water a day, this is 32 ounces. Divide 32 in half, you get 16. Take 16 ounces and divide it by 8, and you get 2. Two ounces of water would be the amount you use for the animal's hourly dose. Once you have determined the right amount of water to use for each dose, add the correct amount of MMS1 your animal should take per hour to this amount of water for his/her dose. Remember, this needs to be calculated according to weight and according to what protocol you are using at the time, as per the charts on pages 301-302.

➤ This may be easier said than done at first. I have used a small syringe for small animals to squirt a dose down the animal's throat. You may know of a better method, and for some animals squirting down the throat may not be good. You want to make absolutely sure you get it down the right pipe and that you do not cause the animal to choke or that you possibly risk asphyxiating them. Please use caution and determine what is the right method for your animal. Also keep in mind you may have to give your animal less water or more water than recommended here. **Be attentive** to what your animal might need.

Explanation of Measurements and Animal Charts

Column Marked Weight of Animal: To use the Dosage Charts for Animals, (pages 301-302), first go to the column marked Weight of Animal. Run your finger down the column to find the weight of the animal, then go across to the column of the protocol you want. Below is a complete explanation of Columns 1 through 6 and what the numbers in each column represents.

Column 1: Starting Procedure dosage for animals. As with humans, always start with the Starting Procedure for animals. The three numbers in this column represent the gradual increase in the dosage. The first number is the starting dose, the second number is the middle dose, and the third number is the maximum dose that you would ever give an animal for that particular weight listed in the column for the Starting Procedure.

Column 2: Protocol 1000 and 1000 Plus dosage for animals. When doing Protocol 1000 for people, you work up gradually to the 3-drop dose; for animals the equivalent to a 3-drop dose is the third figure of the three figures in this column (Column 2). The first number is the starting dose, the second number is the middle dose, and the third number is the maximum dose that you would ever give an animal for that particular weight listed in the column for Protocol 1000.

➤ Always start with the Starting Procedure then move on to Protocol 1000, increasing the dosage slowly to the maximum dose for Protocol 1000, but no higher than the dose listed in Column 2 (Protocol 1000) on the chart for the weight of your animal.

➤ If at any time you notice your animal getting sicker you have increased his dose too quickly. Reduce the dose immediately by 50%. When the sickness passes, gradually build back up to the desired dosage. (See Three Golden Rules for Animals, page 305.)

➤ If the animal does not show signs of improvement after two days, **move on to Protocol 1000 Plus.** This means add DMSO to each oral dose. Continue using the same dosage amounts for Protocol 1000 and add the following amounts of DMSO:

- MMS1 drops—for every 1 drop of MMS1, add 3 drops of DMSO.

- If your animal is small and on Protocol 1000 and the correct dose calls for a fraction of the drop of MMS1, multiply the amount times three. For example, if the dose is 1/2 of a drop of MMS1, three times that amount would be 1 1/2 drops of DMSO. With DMSO you can round the fraction up to the next number. In this case, give 2 drops of DMSO.

- Once you add DMSO to a dose it should be taken within a minute or two at the most.

Column 3: Protocol 2000 dosage for animals. Although Protocol 2000 for people calls for taking MMS1 and MMS2, this column is only for MMS1. This is because normally you would not give an animal MMS2. There are rare exceptions to this however, and I have included details on how to administer MMS2 to animals in Column 4. I have only given two numbers in this column. This is because the principle of Protocol 2000 is you work up to taking as many MMS1 drops as you can per hour but without getting sick (in this case without your animal getting sick).

➤   The first number given in this column (on the row that corresponds to the weight of your animal) is the amount you would begin giving to your animal. This is assuming you have had your animal on Protocol 1000, and worked up to the maximum 3-drop dose equivalent for your animal's weight that Protocol 1000 calls for (as per Column 2). At that point, you start increasing the dosage as is called for in Protocol 2000. If you have not worked up to the equivalent 3-drop dose, then start from whatever dosage you are at and begin gradually increasing the drops in the dose. The second number in this column is the maximum amount of MMS1 that an animal is likely to be able to take according to the animal's weight—never go over the second figure listed.

➤ Start with the first number given in this column, and then increase the amount of MMS1 in small increments after every two to three doses as it seems the animal can take it. Or, if you notice an improvement do not change the dose from that point until there is no more improvement, then you can increase slowly but do not go over the second figure.

➤ If at any time your animal has diarrhea, vomits, or shows other signs of increased sickness, decrease the dosage by 50%. The last amount you gave without the animal getting sicker is most likely the correct dosage, so stick with that amount for some time. If the animal begins to show improvement keep giving the same amount in each dose. If the animal does not show improvement, try increasing the dose gradually. Review the Three Golden Rules of MMS for Animals on page 305.

➤ Remember, on this protocol continue giving DMSO in each dose along with MMS1.

Column 4: MMS2 dosage for animals. MMS2 is difficult with animals and normally you don't have to use MMS2, but if your animal seems resistant to getting better you may want to try it. In that case these are the amounts your animal needs every two hours while on Protocol 2000—the same as with humans. (Read the instructions for Protocol 2000 and adding MMS2 on pages 91-95, and read pages 22-24.) The amounts of MMS2 given in Column 4 of the Animal Dosage Chart 2 (page 302), are the **maximum amounts** to give. Start the animal out with a much smaller dosage than is on the chart and then **work**

up gradually to the amount given. **Do not give any more than this amount 5 times a day,** (separate each MMS2 dose by two hours).

➤ For each milligram (mg) of MMS2 in the capsule (if your animal will swallow a capsule), give 1 milliliter (ml) of water to the animal to wash it down. If the animal wants to drink more water, allow him to drink as much as he wants.

➤ If you are trying capsules and you cannot get the capsule down your animal's throat, you can try putting the MMS2 (calcium hypochlorite) in your animal's drinking water. Determine how much water your animal should drink daily. This is something you can find on the internet. Some say that in general, an animal needs 1 ounce of water per pound of body weight per day. Take the total amount of water your animal is supposed to drink in a day, and add the amount of MMS2 milligrams that your animal should take daily to this drinking water. This would be the dosage amount as listed in Column 4, times 5 (as it is suggested to take 5 doses of MMS2 daily if needed). Remember this would be the maximum dosage to be worked up to, if you are just starting your animal out on MMS2, work up gradually to the amount listed on the chart in Column 4.

➤ If you are serious, you will need to buy a milligram scale. I suggest the Gemini-20 Portable Milligram Scale. It has the capacity to weigh 1 milligram up to 20 grams, which is accurate enough with the capacity for animals weighing from one pound to heavier than a horse. The cost varies from $24.00 USD to $60.00 USD and they can be bought on the internet and shipped almost anywhere in the world. In the US you can buy them from Walmart or online. Go to Google and put in Gemini-20 Portable Milligram scale and you'll find a number of companies that sell this amazing scale. If you don't have a scale and cannot get one, keep in mind that a size #0 capsule holds approximately 300 mg of MMS2 which you could divide several times to get lesser amounts.

Column 5: Protocol 6 and 6 dosage for animals. You may find this column (protocol) the most important and useful because Protocol 6 and 6 will overcome most problems of animals, along with the spray bottle. Just follow the instructions on page 291.

Column 6: MMS1 Maintenance Dosage amounts for animals. A daily maintenance dose of MMS1 can keep your animal clear of toxins, pathogens (sickness causing microorganisms) and parasites. This column indicates the amount of MMS1 your animal should have for daily maintenance, according to weight. Remember, you must mix the MMS1 with water before giving it to your animal.

➤ If you haven't been giving your animal MMS1, and you give him/her a maintenance dose and it makes your animal sick, this is an indication that there are toxins that need to be flushed out. In this case, put your animal on the Starting Procedure, followed by Protocol 1000. After completing Protocol 1000, continue with a daily maintenance dose.

Drinking Water for Animals

Normally, animal's drinking water should be maintained at 1 ppm of chlorine dioxide. This would be 4 MMS1 (activated MMS) drops for each gallon of clean water. Some people have more than one animal and would use this much water in a day, some people may only have one animal and need less water. If you need less water, calculate 1 drop of MMS1, per quart/liter of water.

For those in rural areas or on a farm, slightly turbid water will need more MMS1 per gallon use 6 to 12 drops for

Animal Protocol Dosages: Chart 1

All measurements on this chart are **drops or fractions of drops of MMS1** to be added to the water of the animal's hourly dose.

	1	2	3
Weight of Animal	**Starting Procedure**	**Protocol 1000**	**Protocol 2000**
1 - 2 lbs. (0.45 - 0.9 kg)	1/32–1/16–1/8	1/4–1/4–1/2	1/2–1
2 - 4 lbs (0.9 - 1.8 kg)	1/16–1/6–1/8	1/4–1/4–1/2	3/4–1
4 - 6 lbs (1.8 - 2.7 kg)	1/16–1/8–1/8	1/4–1/4–1/2	3/4–2
6 - 8 lbs (2.7 - 3.6 kg)	1/8–1/8–1/4	1/2–1/2–3/4	1–2
8 - 12 lbs (3.6 - 5.5 kg)	1/8–1/4–1/4	1/2–3/4–1	2–3
12 - 16 lbs (5.5 - 7.2 kg)	1/8–1/4–1/2	1/2–3/4–1	2–3
16 - 22 lbs (7.2 - 10 kg)	1/8–1/4–1/2	1/2–3/4–1	2–4
22 - 30 lbs (10 - 13.6 kg)	1/4–1/2–3/4	1/2–3/4–1	2–4
30 - 40 lbs (13.6 - 18 kg)	1/4–1/2–3/4	3/4–1–1	2–5
40 - 55 lbs (18.1 - 25 kg)	1/4–1/2–3/4	1–1–2	3–5
55 - 75 lbs (25 - 34 kg)	1/4–1/2–3/4	1-1–2	3-6
75 - 100 lbs (34 - 45.4 kg)	1/4–1/2–3/4	1–2–3	4–6
100 - 150 lbs (45.4 - 68 kg)	1/4–1/2–3/4	1–2–3	4–6
150 - 200 lbs (68 - 91 kg)	1/2–3/4–1	1–2–3	4–6
200 - 300 lbs (91 - 136 kg)	1/2–1–2	2–3–6	6–8
300 - 500 lbs (136 - 227 kg)	1–1–2	4–6–10	12–14
500 - 1000 lbs (227 - 454 kg)	2–2–3	8–12–20	25–35
1000 - 1500 lbs (454 - 681 kg)	3–4–5	12–18–30	35–53
1500 - 2300 lbs (681 - 1045 kg)	4–6–8	18–27–45	55–75

Animal Protocol Dosages: Chart 2

The measurements in Column 4 are in **milligrams and grams** as noted. All measurements in Columns 5 and 6 are **drops of MMS1**.

	4	5	6
Weight of Animal	**MMS2 Maximum Dosage**	**6 and 6**	**Daily MMS1 Maintenance**
1 - 2 lbs. (0.45 - 0.9 kg)	2 mg	1 & 1	1
2 - 4 lbs (0.9 - 1.8 kg)	4 mg	1 & 1	1
4 - 6 lbs (1.8 - 2.7 kg)	12 mg	1 & 1	2
6 - 8 lbs (2.7 - 3.6 kg)	16 mg	2 & 2	2
8 - 12 lbs (3.6 - 5.5 kg)	24 mg	3 & 3	3
12 - 16 lbs (5.5 - 7.2 kg)	32 mg	4 & 4	3
16 - 22 lbs (7.2 - 10 kg)	44 mg	4 & 4	4
22 - 30 lbs (10 - 13.6 kg)	60 mg	5 & 5	4
30 - 40 lbs (13.6 - 18 kg)	80 mg	5 & 5	5
40 - 55 lbs (18.1 - 25 kg)	110 mg	6 & 6	5
55 - 75 lbs (25 - 34 kg)	150 mg	6 & 6	6
75 - 100 lbs (34 - 45.4 kg)	200 mg	6 & 6	6
100 - 150 lbs (45.4 - 68 kg)	300 mg	6 & 6	6
150 - 200 lbs (68 - 91 kg)	400 mg	6 & 6	6
200 - 300 lbs (91 - 136 kg)	600 mg	8 & 8	8
300 - 500 lbs (136 - 227 kg)	1 gram	14 & 14	14
500 - 1000 lbs (227 - 454 kg)	2 grams	35 & 35	35
1000 - 1500 lbs (454 - 681 kg)	3 grams	53 & 53	53
1500 - 2300 lbs (681 - 1045 kg)	5 grams	75 & 75	75

slightly turbid water per gallon. The more turbidity the more drops are required. Normally 4 drops of MMS 1 per gallon is plenty.

If you are putting MMS1 in your animal's daily drinking water, this is not enough to serve as a maintenance dose of MMS1. Follow the chart for the daily maintenance dosages for your animal(s) either by putting the dose in their water or giving it to them some other way.

Note: *I suggest using glass or good quality plastic water bowls for your animals if putting MMS in their drinking water. On the other hand, if you **activate MMS first** in a glass or plastic container making it MMS1 and add water, then **after it is activated** and mixed with water it is OK to put in metal containers that are often used for animals. **Do not mix up unactivated MMS (sodium chlorite) and activator directly in a metal bowl or metal cup. First activate and add water in a glass or plastic cup, then put it in the bowl.***

Additional Important Information on How to Administer Certain Protocols to Animals

Protocol 3000 for Animals

Protocol 3000 requires two spray bottles, the same as with humans, one for MMS1 and one for DMSO. To start, wash the area on the animal where you are going to apply the MMS1 and DMSO. Actually it is simple; just spray a leg or area with the amount of MMS1 that it takes to make the liquid reach the skin through the hair. Then spray DMSO on top of that. See below for ideas on how to use a spray bottle for animals. It is OK to mix the two—MMS1 and DMSO—on the body by first spraying one and then spraying the other one on top. **But do not mix MMS1 and DMSO in the same spray bottle** as they will eventually cancel one another out.

Eyes for Animals

Please note, some amounts in this book—such as using MMS1 in the eyes—has been updated since writing my last book. For eyes, I now suggest using a much weaker dosage for animals' eyes—the same protocol as for humans. See pages 136-139 for further explanation and for instructions on mixing up an MMS1 solution for eyes.

Mouth and Teeth for Animals

Use the same measurements and process for brushing the animal's teeth as for people. This will not only help to keep your animal's mouth fresh, but all the same principles apply as for people. Remember, nearly all diseases are influenced to some extent, either large or small, by the condition of the mouth. (See pages 73-76.) It is OK to use the standard spray bottle (see pages 76-77) in your animal's mouth.

Skin Problems for Animals (MMS Spray Bottle)

The number of drops you put in a spray bottle for an animal are the same as for people. However, spraying a hairy animal can be tricky, (for some animals more than others, depending on the length, thickness and amount of hair). If you want the liquid to actually reach the skin, which is the goal, you can accomplish this by parting the hair, spray, and then use your fingers if necessary to lightly pat and help the liquid reach the skin. Then move over another 1/2 inch or so, part the hair again, spray, and so on, until you have covered the entire area needing the spray.

Supporting and Additional Protocols for Animals

For animals, it isn't always easy, but you can use nearly all the other protocols on animals if you need to use them.

Using MMS1 protocols for the eyes, ears, nose, skin problems (spray bottle), the patch, and everything except the oral doses should be the same strength for animals as for people according to the instructions in this book.

Three Golden Rules for Animals

1. If the animal is improving on the dosage you are giving and/or what you are doing, do not change what you are doing—as long as you see improvement, keep it up.

2. The same rule applies for animals as for people: if at any time your animal seems to get sicker on MMS, reduce the dosage you are giving by 50%. Once the sickness passes and the animal is OK with the smaller dosage, you can try to slowly work back up, but be careful to not make the animal sicker.

3. If the animal is not getting better, nor getting worse on the dosage you are giving, **after two or three days,** go to the next higher protocol.

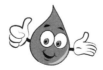

I have been using MMS as a full worming regime for my dogs for about four years with complete success. Keep up the good work. –R.A.

In Conclusion

In closing, remember, nearly all diseases and health problems can be remedied with MMS by following the instructions in this book. I want to say once more, that MMS does not *cure* diseases. MMS kills pathogens and oxidizes poisons anywhere they might be, including in the water of the body. Once pathogens are wiped out and poisons are oxidized, through the normal process of elimination, the body washes them out and then the body is able to heal and be restored to full health.

If you follow these instructions you can regain health in a reasonable amount of time. We encourage you to continue to learn more about how to use MMS. Slot MMS maintenance doses into your daily routine, try to eat real, natural, whole foods, as well as incorporate other healthy practices in your life so that you can reach and maintain optimum health and prevent illness in the future.

Speaking of healthy practices, I want to leave you with perhaps two of the most important *healthy* practices of all time. They are—*always do the right thing*, and *help one another*. Down through the ages, these two concepts have been expressed in varying ways by nearly every ethnic group or religion you can name. That alone should give you a clue—maybe there is merit to living by these standards. Sadly, in today's world they are sometimes grossly overlooked. But I encourage you to adopt these practices as an integral part of your lifestyle. You might just find it makes a huge difference in your happiness and in your health and well-being. If you will *always do the right thing*, and *help one another*, you will reap positive benefits.

Appendix A

CDS, CDH Basic Information

In this book I have chosen to not go into details on either CDS (Chlorine Dioxide Solution) or CDH (Chlorine Dioxide Holding). These are both variations of MMS1, each one requiring a different preparation, although all three are made from the same two ingredients; MMS and an acid activator.

The main goal of this book is to provide a solid foundation of the Health Recovery Plan using MMS1 and MMS2. Once you understand the principles in this book, you can apply them to CDS and CDH, both of which can be used with many MMS protocols.

We are discovering new things about MMS all the time, and about CDS and CDH, which have been around for less time than MMS1. I taught about CDS in my previous book, as well as on instructional videos on YouTube, and about both CDS and CDH in seminars. Since that time, however, some of the information has changed. (So some former teaching and videos are now outdated.) It's an ongoing process. Due to time and space, it is not possible to properly or thoroughly cover CDS and CDH in this book, and as mentioned above, it is important to understand the basic overall principles of MMS and the Health Recovery Plan first. Remember, as with MMS1, always use the Three Golden Rules of MMS (see pages 83-84) if you are using CDS or CDH.

With that said, here is some information regarding some of the differences between CDS, CDH and MMS1.

Over the years I have received a great deal of feedback both from Health Ministers around the world who are very active in helping others recover their health, and from individuals themselves, regarding the three forms of MMS (MMS1, CDS and CDH) and how they have worked for them.

I want to make it clear that we have seen **all forms** of MMS help people recover their health. Nevertheless, there are significant differences with each one. As MMS1 has already been covered extensively in this book, below is a brief synopsis of CDS and CDH.

CDS

CDS was developed by a cattle rancher with direct support and cooperation of Andreas Kalcker. (It was initially developed for use with animals.) CDS is chlorine dioxide gas in distilled water and contains no sodium chlorite or activator. It has to be made up ahead of time through one of several distillation processes and ideally stored in the refrigerator. A pre-made mixture can be convenient. Depending on how CDS is handled, it can last several weeks or even longer.

While CDS is relatively easy to make, there are many variables that can have an effect on the end product. Things such as temperature, climate, altitude, humidity, air pressure, and what type of equipment is used can make a big difference in the resulting CDS. For example, if there is too much air in the bottle or jar it is stored in, it can lose potency. Each time you open the bottle, outgassing occurs which will lessen potency, and so on. Learning the techniques on how to make and handle CDS is not all that difficult if one is dedicated to doing so—but close attention must be given to the details.

CDS is fully activated—there is no residual sodium chlorite left in the solution—which is considered by some to be an advantage. It can be easier on the stomach, and many consider it to have little taste compared to MMS1. At low doses this is true. However, to recover health from serious disease, it is usually necessary to take high level doses of CDS. When this happens, taste and/or burning in the throat can enter into the equation, and sometimes a Herxheimer reaction.

CDS can be helpful for sensitive people, who for one reason or another cannot tolerate MMS1. We have seen that for some people starting out on CDS can be beneficial to help one become accustomed to taking MMS1. The Starting Procedure with MMS1 has eliminated the need for this in most cases. The above stated observations are regarding taking CDS internally. Some people feel that CDS works best with treating external conditions and many have had success with this.

The main important observation that myself and other extensive users of CDS (who have worked close with me) have noticed, is something which I call the *plateau phenomena.* Those working with autistic children used CDS exclusively for one year. At first it was easy to see the children were improving, but as time went on and the children continued to take CDS, the majority seemed to hit a plateau where they were not improving. They came to a standstill. But when these same children were put back on taking MMS1, they again started to improve.

Several Health Ministers and others, when using CDS for a variety of diseases, including cancer, have also reported this phenomenon. There seems to be a point when the individual hits a stalemate (this doesn't always happen, but it often does), but when put on MMS1, they start to improve again. So, if you do use CDS, my advice would be to be aware of the plateau phenomena and if it happens to you, switch to MMS1.

A further word on CDS: There have been differences of opinion over the years regarding the dosing amounts of CDS and the equivalent of CDS to MMS1 for use in our protocols. In the past, we have published a ratio of 1 ml of CDS at 3000 ppm equals a 3-drop dose of MMS1. I have come to believe this is very low dosing for CDS. At the same time, I have come to realize, for multiple reasons too detailed to explain here, that an *exact* equivalent between CDS and MMS1 is not possible to determine.

This is in part due to the reasons mentioned above, the preparation and handling of CDS includes many variables. For example, you may start out with a 3000 ppm solution of CDS, but in a weeks' time, due to out-gassing every time the bottle is opened and other factors, your solution may be getting increasingly weaker. Another reason exact equivalents are difficult to determine is due to the amount of a person's stomach acid. Equivalents can perhaps be determined based on tests with simulated "normal" stomach acid. There are however, many things to consider, one being if the individual indeed does have "normal" stomach acid (most people who have poor health and who are in need of health recovery do not have normal stomach acid). As I have repeatedly said throughout this book, if one follows the Three Golden Rules of MMS, this will indicate if you need to increase or lower your dose.

Probably the most important reason we cannot equate amounts of MMS1 and CDS is that after passing through the stomach, MMS1 still has roughly 50% unactivated sodium chlorite which passes into the human system. Because sodium chlorite has been taken for more than 80 years by hundreds of thousands of people, many of whom swear by it, we must assume that the unactivated sodium chlorite must have some benefit to the system, in addition to the chlorine dioxide. (More on this below.) Since CDS has no sodium chlorite there is no way to make an evaluation of one against the other.

CDH

CDH was developed by Scott McRae and Charlotte Lackney. CDH is also "pre-made" and much easier to make than CDS. It also must be refrigerated. It lasts a couple of weeks to a month in the fridge, depending on the recipe used. CDH, like MMS1, is not totally activated, thus leaving some free sodium chlorite to continue on through the stomach into the system. I have not had extensive experience with CDH, therefore cannot say to use or not use it. We have received reports that it has produced good results for some users.

My Personal Conclusion on MMS1, CDS and CDH

As stated above, CDS is completely activated and contains no residual sodium chlorite in the solution. CDH and MMS1 do contain some free sodium chlorite which makes its way through the stomach into the system. Now, while some people believe the advantage to CDS is that it does not contain unactivated sodium chlorite, I have a different opinion. I believe just the opposite.

Unactivated sodium chlorite alone also destroys poisons and kills pathogens. It has been sold in health food stores in the USA for 80 years and many thousands of people have had some good results from taking it. There are those who now use it without prior activation because they believe that the stomach acid is what activates it and they get a certain amount of good results.

When I first discovered MMS, it was MMS (sodium chlorite) alone that healed the first men in the jungle of malaria. As I traveled throughout the jungle helping many more people recover their health (mostly from malaria and typhoid fever), it was sodium chlorite alone that helped. But the success rate was about 60%. Through much experimentation, it wasn't until I developed the formula further and started activating MMS that the success rate for malaria turned out to be about 98%, and about 92-94% for other diseases.

It is my opinion, unactivated sodium chlorite penetrates deeper into the tissues of the body than even MMS1, according to data I have gleaned from patents issued in the last century. Unactivated sodium chlorite penetrates into the tissues in a different way than MMS1, and thus the two together seem to be more effective than either one alone. **It has been very obvious to many of us that MMS1 (chlorine dioxide) along *with* unactivated sodium chlorite is what gets the very best results.** This is anecdotal evidence, but with many thousands of people recovered, even scientists have to admit that serves as legitimate evidence.

In conclusion, I want to say that MMS in all forms continues to be a mystery at times. The important thing is to find what works best for you. Remember to always use the Three Golden Rules of MMS (pages 83-84). If using CDS or CDH, and you are not seeing desired results, carefully study Chapter 8 in this book and/or consider switching to MMS1.

Appendix B

Genesis II Church of Health and Healing

The Genesis II Church of Health and Healing was formed to serve mankind. To the best of our knowledge the Genesis II Church is the first church ever established with this purpose. The Church now has (as of November 30, 2018) more than 1950 trained Ministers of Health in more than 120 countries. Multitudes of lives have been saved to date, and the suffering of millions has been stopped or adverted.

The word **genesis** in the Church's name signifies *the beginning*. The **number II** signifies bringing about a (new) *second beginning*—it is the intention of the Church to help make a better world. The words **health and healing** signifies that the Church is working towards *bringing health to the world.* The word **church** indicates a *group of people with the same beliefs and purpose concerning serving mankind*.

The purpose of the Church is to help people stay healthy and if they are not, then offer information that they **may** use for themselves and their families, **if they so choose,** to get healthy.

The Genesis II Church of Health and Healing is a non-denominational Church and it welcomes people from all walks of life, religions and belief systems from all other non-violent religions of Earth. The Church does not require that anyone change their beliefs and spiritual practices, but all members are united in the common goal and desire to *help mankind*. The only pre-requisite for becoming a member of the Genesis II Church of Health and Healing is being in support of the following beliefs:

- Doing good deeds
- Good health for all mankind
- Doing what is right
- Freedom for all mankind
- Enlightening others with the truth
- Helping one another
- Living with integrity

Anyone in support of these beliefs is welcome to become a member of the Church.

Jim Humble and Mark Grenon started the Genesis II Church in 2010 in the Dominican Republic. Jim has since retired from the Church and currently the Church is headed up by Mark. Jim continues to work with several MMS projects that he feels are important to complete.

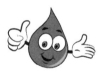

Dog—Gum Growth and Infection: My 12 year old dog had surgery to remove a huge gum overgrowth (epilis) that had overgrown her tooth. After the surgery the site was not healing post-op and looked badly inflamed. After a time another growth was forming in the same spot. Instead of taking her back to the vet I decided to try MMS. I applied MMS to her affected area with a soft toothbrush for a few days and was surprised to find that not only had the inflammation gone away but the new growth had completely vanished. When you look in her mouth there is no sign of anything wrong. It's completely normal.—Elizabeth

Appendix C

Acid-Alkaline Diet

There are many today who promote an alkaline diet. The basic concept is that all diseases live in acid environments and will die when in an alkaline environment. Thus, the idea is that by making your body alkaline, you can kill any disease you have present in your body and live a healthy life. **Just exactly the opposite is true**. This theory lacks scientific facts behind it. The most important basic premise is totally false and can be checked by anyone willing to open their eyes.

Except for the digestive system, the entire human body is alkaline. Most all human diseases exist in the alkaline areas of the body except the digestive system. Most human disease, except for a rare few in the digestive system, are alkaline, not acid. Check out the references listed below.

Alkalinity and acidity in the entire human body are not created by the pH level of the foods one eats. The body uses chemistry to adjust the pH level. Acidity describes the quantity of hydrogen ions in any solution of the body, and alkalinity describes the quantity of hydrogen-oxygen ions in any solution in the body. The body has the total ability to adjust the level of hydrogen ions (acidity), or the level of hydrogen-oxygen ions (alkalinity), anywhere in the body that is required to adjust. The food you eat, or the water you drink has no effect on these levels, that is, until you overdo them so far that you become sick.

There are probably more than 100 web sites that promote the alkaline diet. Many of them sell alkaline water. Your body must maintain a low alkaline condition everywhere except the digestive system. Every organ of the body has a different alkaline level in order for the body to function properly. Your blood is maintained at 7.41 pH for arteries and 7.3 pH for veins. That's alkaline not acid, and it cannot be changed. Nowhere in the body can you change these exact alkaline or pH levels. Drinking alkaline water of 9.5 pH just makes the body work harder to get rid of the extra alkalinity, which the body naturally does. When your urine turns alkaline that merely means that the body is off-loading the alkalinity that it doesn't need. It does not mean you are healthy.

The alkaline [diet] theory web sites say you must eat alkaline forming fruits and vegetables, but nearly all fruits and vegetables are acidic. When you put acidic fruits and vegetables in your stomach, the stomach increases the acidity by adding hydrochloric acid, but when those fruits and vegetables go from the stomach to the intestine the body releases an enzyme that makes them all alkaline. Nothing escapes this function of the body. No alkaline food or alkaline water can change that.

Here is a list put out by the FDA of more than 200 vegetables, fruits, meats, and other foods—showing that all these foods are acidic. Remember, anything below 7 pH is acidic, and over 7 pH is alkaline. Check it out:

http://webpal.org/SAFE/aaarecovery/2_food_st orage/Processing/lacf-phs.htm

I can't debunk all the various cancer treatments that don't work, nor list all those that have been known to work. But I mention the alkaline theory here as many thousands of people are getting the wrong data from dozens, maybe as many as 100 web sites.

The links below are web sites telling facts you can check, telling the truth about the acid-alkaline theory of diseases.

The pH of blood. On the internet go to Google or any search engine and put in the search "pH of blood". You will get many answers but they will all be the same.

https://sciencebasedpharmacy.wordpress.com/2 009/11/13/your-urine-is-not-a-window-to-your-body-ph-balancing-a-failed-hypothesis/
This is a complete explanation of why you cannot change your body pH. Each pH area is solidly in place and does not balance against other pH's of the body. Very good explanation.

http://www.chemistry.wustl.edu/~edudev/LabT utorials/Buffer/Buffer.html
Acid-Base Equilibra Experiment, by Rachel Casiday and Regina Frey, Department of Chemistry, Washington University St. Louis, MO 63130.

http://wikipedia.org/wiki/blood
Blood – Wikipedia, the free encyclopedia.

http://curezone.com/forums/fm.asp?i=840037
Digestive System and pH Level. This article is well documented giving 24 research papers showing pH level of the entire digestive system and it shows that the stomach is highly acid and the small upper intestine is alkaline.

http://en.wikipedia.org/wiki/PH
pH of *body* fluids, and *organs* are tightly regulated in a process called acid-base homeostasis. You can't change the pH of the body.

http://www.ncbi.nlm.nih.gov/pubmed/16277975
Alkaline pH Homeostasis in Bacteria: New Insights. Shows that pathogenic bacteria (disease causing) survives in alkaline environment.

http://textbookofbacteriology.net/nutgro_4.html
Please note that neutrophiles are hard to find because the spelling only adds an "e" at the end of the word neutrophil, but this is the link to one of many web sites explaining neutropiles as disease causing microbes. There are 210 neutroppiles that are disease causing living at an alkaline pH.

http://en.wikipedia.org/wiki/Alkaline diet
More acid-alkaline theory.

http://www.clinchem.org/content/41/10/1522.full.pdf
Composition of interstitial fluid. Regulation of pH to 7.3 to 7.4.

http://articles.mercola.com/sites/articles/archive/2010/09/11/alkaline-water-interview.aspx
Article: Alkaline Water: If You Fall for This "Water Fad" You Could Do Some Major Damage.

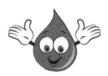

Cat—Eye Herpes: My cat had crusty eyes all the time. The vet would prescribe ointment for her eyes when it got bad, but other than that she said there wasn't anything they could do. It was a form of herpes in the cat's eyes, probably passed on from the mom cat. I had to wipe her eyes with a damp cloth every day. I mixed one drop of activated MMS with water and squirted it in her mouth daily. She didn't like it, but she didn't throw it up either. Within two weeks her eyes cleared up and remained clear...I'm glad she didn't have crusty, weepy eyes anymore!—Sunni, United States

Links of Interest

This book is the latest official information from Jim Humble about MMS as of January 2019.

For More Information:

https://jimhumble.co/
https://mmstestimonials.co/
https://www.mmswiki.is/

Contact:

healthrecovery@jimhumble.is

Jim Humble Books:

https://www.jhbooks.org

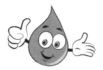

Flu: If I told you there was an anti-viral you could prepare in your kitchen to prevent the flu in a day, would you believe me? My daughter woke up crying yesterday morning with a 104 degree fever and chills not to mention the nausea and headache. Poor girl. It was time to kick into healing mode for her. We both took about 5 doses of MMS yesterday. Twenty-four hours later she is fever free and I never got sick.—H.P., Arizona

❧

Asthma: After using MMS my asthma was gone in 2 days flat, never to return. I also use MMS when I feel a cold coming up, and for the last 2 years I never had a cold again. MMS stops it in its tracks. —Monika

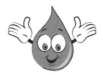

Chronic Fatigue: I took MMS for about two and a half weeks and I have to say I'm very intrigued. I have dealt with chronic fatigue for many years and have tried a lot of different things but I felt like this started having some positive effects very quickly. I had had a blocked nose for months and within a couple of days of taking the drops my nose was clear and I felt like I had more energy. My concentration is also significantly improved. On the whole I'm feeling a lot better than what I did before...Thanks very much for taking the time to provide this 'stuff' for those that are in need of something effective to help them with their health issues. —Richie

Lung Cancer: I have my own testimony for the treatment of lung cancer. I have my own medical diagnosis "Inter DiaCor". Having problems with sweating, dry cough, fatigue, nervousness, severe pain in the middle of the back, hard to sleep and pain when lying on the left side, I decided to do a complete analysis of the organism. I found a great contamination of bacteria and viruses in each lung, but mostly on the left. Also found a weak and small alveolar gas exchange. I started using MMS Protocol 1000. Control analysis: I have worked for 15 days and the result was 50% less microorganism, still I continued with MMS. I've done the analysis after 30 days and the result was 100% clean lungs. I continued to drink MMS for 20 days due to parasites in the cerebral cortex, the brain, and by the end I was able to repair all the problems in 52 days. Initially, the viral load was 86.1%, and finally 4.6%. I have all the images of such evidence. I have other people with bone cancer, severe toxemia, depression and the like. The success for these came in 30 days. This is truly amazing! —B.T., Croatia

MMS Helped My Herpes/Vaginosis/Yeast Infection: I was diagnosed with Herpes about four months ago and that was probably the hardest news for me to hear...I knew my dad was taking MMS for other health reasons, but I had no clue about what all the amazing things that MMS could help your body fight off. My dad bought me the book and a couple of bottles of MMS to get me started. I am happy and proud to say that I got a blood test two months later and I tested negative. I didn't take it for two months, I followed the protocol, but it took me about two months to get the courage to see if what I had done worked. I am amazed by MMS and the issues that it helps your body with. When I was dealing with herpes, I also had bacterial vaginosis and a yeast infection, all of which cleared up. —Gage, United States

Alzheimer's Gone: I am familiar with Alzheimer's, so when I had symptoms occur, they were familiar to me. I noticed I was not coping socially, and I was starting to have total gaps in my memory (and thus withdrawing). Because I had heard of MMS being used to cure dementia I decided I had nothing to lose. I followed the protocol for one month, slowly building up to the full dose of 3 drops every hour for 8 hours, and staying with the regime, for the full period, (it is important to note that if the dose is causing you to feel unwell, cut back on the doses per day and keep it low for 2 days then start to increase to the level you can tolerate, but do not stop all together). By the end of the treatment I noticed a remarkable change in my cognition, and as time goes on my condition continues to improve. I feel like a new person, I am social again, happy, and look forward to each new day. —Sam

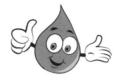

Sinus Infection: I have had a sinus condition for years. My sinuses were always blocked up, particularly in the morning. I also got blood in the tissues fairly often when I blew my nose to relieve the blockages. Initially I was taking MMS because I was always hungry and because of that over weight. This was just a just a shot in the dark after reading other peoples success stories. The results of my taking MMS was that my consistent hunger went away and to my surprise the sinus condition also went away. I have had the sinus condition for so long that it seemed normal. In hindsight I believe both were caused by candida. —Chris, United States

ॐ

Stage 4 Cancer: In March, an 80 year old man was diagnosed with cancer stage 4. I witnessed the medical consult and the man was told he had only two/three months to live. I told the man I could help him and started the MMS1 protocol for cancer stage 4. After two weeks taking MMS1 he felt much better and began to gain weight again. He also started taking MMS2 four times a day. Today, April 30th, he feels better than ever before and gained over 10 pounds weight! He should be dead by now, but no way thanks to MMS1 and MMS2. —Robert

ॐ

Hepatitis C: Two years ago I was diagnosed with Hep C. I used MMS for a little over a month and my readings are now fine. As an added benefit, my lungs became clear, multiple skin conditions and additional virus' are gone, brown teeth turned white and white hair turned brown. God Bless You, Jim. —J.M., United States

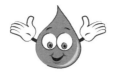

Arthritis in Wrist Gone: I have known of MMS for years, but not the protocol for cancer. I started using the cancer protocol for a 21 year old malignant breast tumor this year without knowing about the protocol for arthritis. To my amazement, the arthritis in my left wrist and hand has disappeared. I got on the website and lo and behold others had been using it with success for arthritis as well. One of the points I would like to make here is that I was not influenced in any way by others reports. The pain of arthritis may not be life threatening, but it certainly takes away from life enjoyment. Thank you Jim Humble. —Judith E., United States

Crohn's Disease: I've had Crohn's for four years. I took MMS for one week, and my symptoms abated. I quit taking my medication to see what would happen. I have been fine ever since. —R.W., United States

Systemic Candida: For years I have had a problem with feeling sick after vigorous exercise. It has gotten progressively worse over time. I suspected systemic Candida, but was never diagnosed. I tried Protocol 1000 and added DMSO. Three weeks later I was ready to test the effectiveness of this treatment. I have exercised extremely hard for the past two weeks, with appropriate breaks, and I feel terrific! I have had no indication of my former problems. By the way I am 72 years old, but now feel like I'm in my 20's. MMS really worked for me. —Richard

NOTES

About the Author

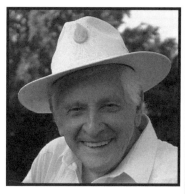

Jim Humble first began his work in the health field in his early 20's when he became the manager of a health food store in Los Angeles, California. He authored a 200 question "Nutritional Evaluation Test" that determined the vitamins, minerals, proteins, and fats a person's body might be deficient in. The test was later computerized and was considered by many to be the most accurate method of determining deficiencies known at the time. Over the years Jim has maintained his interest in alternative health, and worked with numerous healing modalities including healing his own broken neck in record time using magnets. He has authored many successful books and his current developments are outlined in this instruction guidebook.

Jim first started his career in the Aerospace industry, where he quickly became a research engineer. He worked on the first intercontinental missile, wrote instruction manuals for the first vacuum tube computers, worked on secret radio control electronics, and dozens of other "state of the art" electronic projects at Hughes Aircraft Company, Northrop Aircraft, General Motors Research Defense Laboratories, and others.

After 20 years in the Aerospace Industry, Jim went into gold mining where he developed methods of gold recovery that replace the use of mercury to help overcome health issues for small miners. He wrote 5 books on the subject of recovering gold from its ores. In 1996, while prospecting for gold in South America, he discovered what has come to be known as MMS, a simple health formula that eradicates malaria. In the years that followed, he worked to further improve the formula. Eventually a missionary group invited him to Africa where he successfully helped over 5,000 malaria cases and victims of other diseases recover their health. Since that time, hundreds of thousands of people have used MMS to recover their health from a wide range of diseases.

For more information:
https://jimhumble.co/
https://mmstestimonials.co/
https://www.mmswiki.is/

Contact: *healthrecovery@jimhumble.is*